THE
ULTIMATE
PCOS HANDBOOK

Also by Colette Harris and Theresa Cheung

The PCOS Diet Book
You Can Beat PMS

THE ULTIMATE PCOS HANDBOOK

LOSE WEIGHT, BOOST FERTILITY, CLEAR SKIN AND RESTORE SELF-ESTEEM

**COLETTE HARRIS
& THERESA CHEUNG**

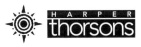

HARPER thorsons

10% OF AUTHOR ROYALTIES GO TO
VERITY, THE PCOS CHARITY

HarperThorsons
An Imprint of HarperCollins*Publishers*
77–85 Fulham Palace Road
Hammersmith, London W6 8JB

The website address is: www.thorsonselement.com

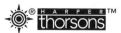

and *HarperThorsons* are trademarks of
HarperCollins*Publishers* Ltd

First published by HarperThorsons 2006

10 9 8 7 6 5 4

A catalogue record of this book is
available from the British Library

ISBN-13 978-0-00-721325-2
ISBN-10 0-00-721325-5

Printed and bound in Great Britain by
Martins the Printers, Berwick-upon-Tweed

CONTENTS

PART THREE: TAKING CHARGE OF PCOS: Nurturing Your Emotions and Spirit

INTRODUCTION:
TAKING CONTROL

Writing this book in 2006, we're delighted to see that the void in patient information about PCOS that existed 10 years ago is slowly being filled, and the condition is more readily recognized and diagnosed by doctors. When Colette's first book *The Woman's Guide to PCOS* was published in 2000, it was the first guide for women coping with the condition, and it was a struggle to get interest from newspapers, TV or the medical community, but slowly and surely we did just that.

With the fantastic rise of websites, from Verity in the UK to PCOSupport in the US and Australia, and chat rooms where women from all over the world can share their thoughts and questions, the world of PCOS in 2006 is a very different place. Even celebrities with PCOS have finally come forward and increased media interest.

Yet many of us still feel that PCOS is taking over our lives and emotions and leaving us feeling out of control, as these quotes from women like us show:

'Some days when my symptoms flare up I find it hard to leave the house. How could I with hair sprouting on my chin, a bloated stomach and acne breaking out? On days like that people have no idea how tough it is for me even to do routine things, like shopping or running errands.'

'This thing is so hard to deal with. Not only is it impossible for me to lose weight but I'm finding it hard to get pregnant. I got married a few years ago, and whenever people ask why we're delaying starting a family and I tell them I've got PCOS, their eyes glaze over.'

'The symptoms of PCOS strike at the heart of my femininity; they attack the very heart of who and what I am. I'm always tired and my libido is non-existent. I can't imagine why any man would want to cuddle up to me.'

And this is backed up by research – here's an extract from a recent study into the psychology of PCOS:

Previous research on polycystic ovarian syndrome (PCOS) has overwhelmingly been conducted within a medical or psychiatric framework, and has failed to explore women's own experience of the syndrome. Interviews were conducted with 30 women with PCOS recruited through a national self-help organization. Thematic analysis of the interviews revealed pervasive reports of feeling 'freakish', 'abnormal', and not 'proper' women. These feelings were related to three symptoms commonly experienced by women with PCOS: 'excess' hair growth, irregular, absent or disrupted periods, and infertility. Smooth hairless bodies and faces, regular menstruation and the capacity to bear children were associated with femininity, and as a result of their symptoms women expressed feeling 'different' from other women and less 'feminine'. The results are discussed and it's suggested that polycystic ovarian syndrome is a deeply stigmatizing condition, 'a theft of womanhood', with far-reaching implications for all women, whether or not they conform to 'feminine' norms.[1]

Other research[2] confirms the seriousness of the emotional impact that PCOS can have on the quality of everyday life and our love lives.

In other words, PCOS isn't just about your ovaries or your medical tests. It's about the whole of you – mind, body and spirit.

Whether you're dealing with weight issues, struggling with facial hair, feeling frustrated with fertility, having the odd sensation that you just don't feel quite right, or worrying about your increased risk of diabetes or heart disease, there's little doubt that having PCOS can prevent you from wholeheartedly embracing your life. It can make you feel swamped. And the fact that there's no magic 'cure' can leave you feeling overwhelmed.

That's why we decided to write *The Ultimate PCOS Handbook*. We've both got PCOS ourselves, and have found that there's nothing like fighting back to help you feel better about yourself, better about life, and better physically as your self-help strategies help your symptoms recede.

If you've ever sought medical help, and been made to feel you're fussing about nothing, or that you should just take the Pill, go away and come back for more drug treatment when you want to get pregnant, this book's for you.

If you've ever tried to explain your condition to a friend, relative or co-worker, and they've looked at you like you're from another planet, then read on!

If you've ever found yourself thinking 'Why me? Haven't I got enough to cope with?' or you've felt frustrated that this feeling of powerlessness is sapping your confidence and eating away at your *joie de vivre*, it's time to say 'No' to PCOS ruling your life.

This ultimate handbook shows you all the things you can do to take control of your symptoms, your health and your happiness, starting from today. Whether it's boosting your understanding of your condition so you can talk to your medical practitioner with more confidence, discovering the best foods to eat to help you lose weight or boost fertility, or working out how a lifestyle and exercise plan can enhance your medication, you'll find it all here, plus inspiring thoughts and stories from other women who have taken charge of their PCOS and transformed their lives as a result.

We've both used the information and ideas in this book to get our health and our lives back on track (read our success stories on page 353), and we hope it helps you to choose a positive, happier, healthier future, and create a sense of yourself, not as a woman ruled or defined by her PCOS, but as a woman living a fulfilling life who just happens to deal with PCOS along with the bills, the laundry, the kids, the job, the whole kit and kaboodle.

We hope you find taking charge of your PCOS using this handbook to be a satisfying, revitalizing experience. Good luck! And don't forget to pass on your success stories to other women with PCOS too.

Colette and Theresa
January 2006

PART ONE
THE LOW-DOWN ON PCOS

CHAPTER I
WHAT EXACTLY IS PCOS?

Polycystic ovary syndrome (PCOS) is a metabolic disorder that disrupts your hormones, typically giving you higher-than-normal levels of certain sex hormones and insulin, which can trigger symptoms such as irregular (or no) periods, acne, excess hair and weight gain. You may also have a number of cysts on your ovaries – these show up as dark blobs on an ultrasound scan. These are in fact empty egg follicles in a state of 'suspended animation', waiting for the right balance of sex hormones to come along and activate them. About one in 10 women in the UK, US and Australia develops the condition.[1]

Most women with PCOS start to notice symptoms in their late teens or twenties. There's a range of symptoms,[2] but you're likely to have one or more of the following:

- absent, infrequent or irregular periods due to the imbalance of hormones

- subfertility, as you need to ovulate to become pregnant and some women with PCOS don't ovulate regularly or at all
- acne which lasts longer than the normal teenage years – this happens if you produce too much testosterone
- obesity or weight gain
- insulin resistance: a higher-than-normal amount of insulin in your body, which creates an imbalance with other hormones and puts you at increased risk of Type 2 diabetes (by up to 40 per cent by age 40)
- excess hair (hirsutism) – if you produce too much testosterone – which can develop in places such as the face, chest and tummy
- alopecia (thinning hair) particularly at the top of your head and on your temples if you produce too much testosterone
- Long-term health risks.[3] Women with PCOS tend to have a higher-than-normal risk of developing diabetes and a high cholesterol level later in life. It also increases your risk of having a stroke and developing uterine cancer.

HOW TO GET A DIAGNOSIS

If you suspect that you've got PCOS, you'll need to see your doctor. If your GP also suspects that you have PCOS, they may refer you to a hospital specialist in endocrinology (medicine relating to hormones) or a gynaecologist (a specialist in women's reproductive systems and hormones).

There are ways[4] to confirm if you have PCOS:

1. Talking to your GP: your doctor will look out for typical symptoms such as menstrual disturbance, hyperinsulinaemia or insulin resistance (we'll discuss this in more detail later on), hair and skin problems, and obesity. These aren't foolproof indications, however, as you can have other symptoms, too. For instance, though many women with PCOS have irregular or absent periods, and many have menstrual cycle lengths greater than 35 days, you can still have PCOS even if your cycles are regular. And only around 40–60 per cent of women with PCOS are obese,[5] so you may not be overweight. There's also a distinct group of thin PCOS patients who may have even more firmly entrenched hormonal and fertility problems than their obese counterparts. And not all patients are excessively hairy but may have other problems such as acne. So your doctor can do medical tests, too.

2. Laboratory testing: Blood tests measure the levels of certain hormones so that a diagnosis of PCOS can be made. There's considerable disagreement in the medical community about which tests to use, but generally the following are tested: FSH (follicle-stimulating hormone), LH (luteinizing hormone), total testosterone, sex hormone-binding globulin, prolactin, thyroid-stimulating hormone, fasting insulin and glucose levels. These are best obtained in the first 2–3 days after the onset of a period. A blood lipid profile should be part of every evaluation, as should a glucose tolerance test and a test to measure insulin levels.

3. Ultrasound scan: Transvaginal ultrasound[6] is a way for your pelvis and ovaries to be 'mapped' to see if your ovaries look as if they are affected by PCOS. A hand-held probe is inserted directly into the vagina to scan the pelvic structures, while ultrasound pictures are viewed on a

monitor. The test can be performed to evaluate women with infertility problems, abnormal bleeding, sources of unexplained pain and to diagnose PCOS by looking for slight enlargement of the ovaries and the empty follicles that show up as black 'blobs' on the scan (see diagram on page 9).

HOW DOES PCOS AFFECT MY OVARIES?

You have two ovaries, small organs inside your body where the egg cells are produced and stored. At puberty the number of fully-formed cells is around 300,000 – and when your body's reproductive system is activated by puberty's cascade of sex hormones, pumped into your bloodstream by the ovaries and adrenal glands, then each month about 20 of these egg cells, each encased in a sac called a follicle, begin to mature. One follicle eventually becomes dominant while the others shrink away. The egg within the dominant follicle continues ripening to maturity, then exits the ovary and enters the adjacent fallopian tube either to be fertilized or, if conception doesn't happen, expelled from the body during menstruation.

But this normal cycle relies on a complex web of hormones being present at the right time, in the right amounts, for ovulation to happen. Having PCOS often interferes with this, affecting your ovaries' abilities to nurture, mature and release an egg each month.

The best way to get to grips with how your ovaries are affected by PCOS is to compare a 'normal' menstrual cycle with a typical PCOS cycle.

THE NORMAL MENSTRUAL CYCLE

The length of the menstrual cycle can vary from a short 21 days to a long cycle of 40 days. The length of the cycle is calculated by counting the first day of bleeding as Day 1 and then counting until the very last day before the next bleed (period). The average menstrual cycle is commonly described as 28 days, although this may be true for only one in 10 women.

In a normal menstrual cycle lasting approximately 28 days, the first half (called the follicular phase) starts on the first day of your period and lasts for about 14 days. In this phase the pituitary gland releases low levels of FSH (follicle-stimulating hormone) to stimulate the follicles in the ovary to ripen their eggs and produce the hormone oestrogen, which causes the lining of the womb to start to thicken in preparation for pregnancy. When levels of oestrogen are high enough, the pituitary gland produces a large amount of LH (luteinizing hormone) and the dominant matured follicle in the ovary releases its egg into the fallopian tubes towards the womb.

After ovulation comes the second stage of the menstrual cycle, called the luteal phase. Here the cells from the burst follicle collapse to form a 'cyst', or new kind of follicle, called the *corpus luteum*. The corpus luteum now produces progesterone as the main hormone of the second half of the cycle. Progesterone causes the thickened lining of the womb to secrete nutrients ready to receive the fertilized egg. If the egg is fertilized by a sperm following intercourse it will implant itself in the womb lining, and the corpus luteum will continue to grow to protect the pregnancy. If it isn't fertilized 14 days after ovulation, the corpus luteum stops producing progesterone and oestrogen. The thickened womb lining breaks down and is shed as a period, ready for the whole cycle to start again.

WHAT HAPPENS DURING A PCOS CYCLE?

The diagram opposite shows a normal menstrual cycle compared to a PCOS cycle. With PCOS, LH levels are often high when the menstrual cycle starts. The levels of LH are also higher than FSH levels. Because the LH levels are already quite high, the surge that sets off the chain-reaction causing ovulation doesn't happen. Without this LH surge, ovulation doesn't occur and periods are irregular.

WHAT DOES A POLYCYSTIC OVARY LOOK LIKE?

Polycystic means 'many cysts' and gives the condition its name, but in actual fact in PCOS, the word 'cyst' simply means an empty egg follicle. A polycystic ovary usually has 8 to 12 or more cysts on its surface. Each cyst measures 2–9 mm in size (see diagram opposite).

A cyst is a fluid-filled sac, and in PCOS that means the empty follicles that are in 'suspended animation' – not given the right hormones in the right amounts at the right time. If you've got polycystic ovaries the follicles may stop growing too early, preventing the release of an egg. Instead of bursting to release the egg, they gradually build up on the ovaries to form lots of small cysts which are actually swollen egg chambers waiting for the right hormone to trigger the maturation and release of an egg.

There's a characteristic pattern of ovarian enlargement to 1.5 to 3 times normal size, and a number of small cystic structures of less than 10 mm, which are usually located in a circle around the ovarian surface, commonly called a 'string of pearls'.

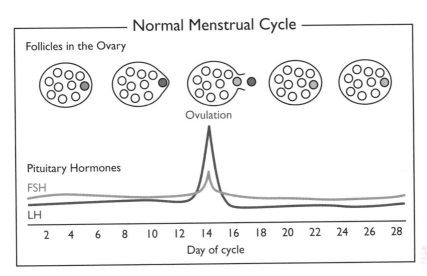

Normal Menstrual Cycle

Follicles in the Ovary

Ovulation

Pituitary Hormones

FSH

LH

2   4   6   8   10   12   14   16   18   20   22   24   26   28

Day of cycle

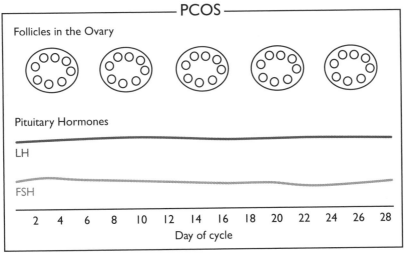

PCOS

Follicles in the Ovary

Pituitary Hormones

LH

FSH

2   4   6   8   10   12   14   16   18   20   22   24   26   28

Day of cycle

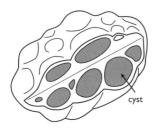

cyst

Polycystic Ovary

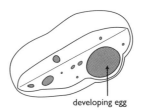

developing egg

Normal Ovary

DOES PCOS MEAN I HAVE OVARIAN CYSTS?

Ovarian cysts are a common but usually unrelated gynaecological disorder. They differ from polycystic ovaries in that they 1) are typically found *within* the ovary 2) they occur singly and not in groups and 3) can, if left untreated, become cancerous. Polycystic ovaries, on the other hand, are neither cancerous nor are they likely to become so.

WHAT CAUSES PCOS?

PCOS continues to perplex even the medical experts[7] who specialize in it. We know that there's a very strong genetic and hereditary basis of PCOS,[8] but even if two women have the same gene they may end up with different symptoms, depending on their environment and lifestyle.

⇨ TIME FOR A NAME CHANGE?

As the 'cysts' in PCOS aren't actually cysts at all, and because a woman who's had her ovaries removed can still have PCOS symptoms, some scientists are calling for a name change for the condition – if the underlying metabolic condition affects your ovaries, then your ovaries aren't the cause and shouldn't be the main focus of the name.

'Polyfollicular syndrome' has been suggested, as have 'ovarian dysmetabolic syndrome', 'Syndrome O', 'cystic ovaries', 'functional hyper-androgenism', 'Stein-Leventhal syndrome' and 'chronic anovulation'.

It's fantastic that the condition has become a talking point among medical specialists, and while PCOS may be an imperfect name, whatever the syndrome is eventually called, it matters most that it's recognized, evaluated and treated.

The effect of environment and lifestyle is also clear because you can have polycystic ovaries (PCO) without having the syndrome (PCOS).

With pelvic ultrasound it has been found that approximately 20–30 per cent of women of reproductive age will have polycystic ovaries, but only about half of these will have the signs or symptoms of PCOS. If the otherwise 'normal' group is examined closely, experts[9] believe they may be experiencing the subtle hormonal changes associated with PCOS, but just have them under control, perhaps due to diet, exercise and lifestyle factors. But women with PCO are thought to be predisposed to develop PCOS if those lifestyle factors change, and if they do it could have a significant impact on their long-term health, such as an increased risk of diabetes and heart disease.

It's also possible to have PCOS symptoms but *not* have polycystic ovaries on a scan. This makes sense if you think that the ovarian changes are just another symptom of the underlying cause of PCOS – which we'll talk about in the next chapter.

'When I was finally diagnosed with PCOS the relief was incredible. Knowing what is wrong with me gives me choices.'
Susan, 38

CHAPTER 2
WHAT CAUSES PCOS?

The search for the underlying cause of PCOS is ongoing. Here's what researchers have uncovered so far.

IT'S ALL IN THE GENES!

Researchers have noticed that PCOS tends to run in families, and a number of studies[1] suggest that genes play a part in developing the syndrome. A gene is a basic unit of heredity; bits of DNA that direct the reproduction, growth and function of cells. Symptoms are fairly easy to track down through the generations. There may be early male-pattern baldness in men (where the hairline recedes at the front and on the crown) and PCOS symptoms in women. The long-term health risks of PCOS – such as diabetes, high blood pressure and obesity – can also be seen in both sexes, and it's thought that if a woman has PCOS, then her immediate family members have a 50–50 chance of having it too.

⇨ CAN GUYS HAVE PCOS?

Some researchers believe that the PCOS gene can be passed down in men as well as women. Obviously it's harder to diagnose in men, because they don't have ovaries and don't have periods, and what would be considered hirsutism (excess hair) in women would be considered normal hair distribution in men. Still, a number of different findings have suggested a pattern of symptoms which, if found together, may represent the male counterpart of PCOS:

- Increased number of hair follicles
- Low sperm count
- Premature balding
- Insulin resistance
- Weight gain in the stomach area
- Increased risk of diabetes and heart disease.

All this is currently speculative, but the signs that link some aspects of PCOS to male relations[2] of women with PCOS adds weight not only to the pattern of inheritance theory but also to the ongoing argument against the appropriateness of the current name for the broad spectrum of symptoms associated with PCOS.

PCOS also seems to be more common among women from southern Asia than in white Caucasian women, but no one yet knows why.

Researchers are currently using gene technology to try and discover if any specific genes trigger PCOS. They need several hundred families to take part and the process can take decades. So far, studies that have concentrated on genes controlling oestrogen and progesterone have found no genetic link. But an interesting 1997 study[3] showed that in PCOS a faulty gene may be involved in the first stage of testosterone production, and could account for the raised levels of this hormone often seen in women with PCOS. It's possible that this gene may interact with other genes and with the environment to produce PCOS. Another study[4] revealed that there may be a link between a specific variation in the insulin gene and the failure to ovulate in women with PCOS.

Other research suggests that PCOS may represent the final outcome of different, deeply inter-related genetic abnormalities and environmental factors that influence each other and perpetuate the syndrome.[5] Most women dealing with the condition believe this to be true. We all know that if we're stressed or put on weight or don't exercise, it affects our symptoms.

Research into the genetics of PCOS continues – but what's in it for us? If we can discover what genes trigger the syndrome, medical companies hope to develop medicines based on this knowledge, and perhaps even tests that can show very early on in life whether a person has PCOS or not, so you could create a diet and lifestyle to combat the problem, right from the start.

'The biochemistry of PCOS is fascinating – but even more gripping is the realization that here is a genetic condition where, although there is no cure, sufferers can control the outcome through diet and lifestyle,' says Dr Adam Carey, reproductive endocrinologist and nutritionist. 'It is a condition where women really can use their environment to interact with their genetic programming and create a positive outcome.'

TOO MUCH MALE HORMONE?

Another theory about what causes PCOS is that women with the condition produce too much testosterone – a hormone known as the 'male' hormone because men produce 10 times more than women. In PCOS, the excess testosterone finds its way into the body's circulation and triggers the familiar PCOS symptoms of hair loss, facial hair and acne. Testosterone can also be converted into oestrogen in the fat stores of the body. The result: weight gain and hormonal havoc.

It appears that a malfunction with the hypothalamus–pituitary regulation of the menstrual cycle in women with PCOS causes the release of abnormal levels of hormones, in particular testosterone. Not only do high levels of luteinizing hormone (LH) stimulate the production of testosterone in the ovaries, but when the ovaries aren't working as they should they become thickened, and this thickening produces even more testosterone.

Several studies have linked excess androgens (male hormones, including testosterone) with PCOS. Testosterone is the most often cited, but research[6] has also suggested that PCOS may be the result of a surge of another male hormone, adrenal androgen DHEA. DHEA is responsible for the production of pubic and armpit hair in puberty. This has yet to be proved conclusively, but it's interesting as many women with PCOS date the beginning of their problems from puberty, when male hormones first surge.

'I was 15 when I first noticed something was wrong. My friends had mild acne, but my face exploded. My friends started their periods, but I didn't.'
Laura, 21

Some experts believe that even you haven't got high levels of testosterone you may become more sensitive to it if you have PCOS, and go on to develop symptoms associated with testosterone excess because of that sensitivity, rather than increased levels. This could explain why some women with PCOS don't show high testosterone levels in blood tests, even though they have the symptoms.

Testosterone is carried in the bloodstream by a protein called sex hormone-binding globulin (SHGB). Higher-than-normal insulin levels in the bloodstream can suppress the production of SHBG so that the amount of unbound (active) testosterone is raised – the reason why some women with high insulin levels (common if you're overweight) can have signs of testosterone excess even when tests reveal a normal level in the blood.

▷ HOW MUCH IS TOO MUCH?

The normal blood testosterone level in women should be around 0.5–3.5 nmol per litre (a small measure of a substance in a solution); in men usually 15–30 nmol per litre. Women with PCOS tend to have a testosterone level of 2.5–5.0 nmol per litre. If the level goes higher than 5.0 nmol then other problems such as congenital adrenal hyperplasia and ovarian tumours need to be ruled out.

Mild testosterone excess in women can cause symptoms such as acne, hirsutism and alopecia (thinning hair on the head) and these symptoms are often called androgenization or hyperandrogenism. It's important to point out, though, that testosterone levels in women with PCOS don't usually get so high as to cause a condition called virilization, which is when the voice gets deeper, breasts shrink and the clitoris enlarges.

TOO MUCH LH?

High blood levels of the pituitary hormone LH are also commonly found in women with PCOS, and higher-than-normal LH levels can trigger the production of testosterone and the familiar symptoms of PCOS.[7]

The high levels of LH may be due to lack of ovulation, as both oestrogen and progesterone inhibit the production of LH, but some women with PCOS and regular ovulations also have high LH levels, indicating that in some cases there may be a problem with the pituitary gland itself or with its ability to interact with the ovaries.

BLAME IT ON THE INSULIN!

In the last few years, research[8,9] has discovered that a condition known as *insulin resistance* plays an important role in the cause of PCOS. Major reviews on the subject suggest that up to 70 per cent of women with PCOS who are overweight can have insulin resistance, and around 30 per cent of women who are slim can have it, too.

Women with insulin resistance have raised levels of insulin in their bloodstream, and high levels of insulin have been shown to stimulate the ovaries to produce more testosterone and lower blood levels of SHBG, resulting in higher and more active levels of testosterone.

'I only found out I had insulin resistance as well as PCOS when I got pregnant. Tests revealed that my blood sugar levels were all over the place.'
Alice, 36

⇨ WHAT IS INSULIN RESISTANCE?

Insulin is a powerful hormone released by your pancreas in response to eating food – especially carbohydrates. It transports sugar out of the blood and into muscle, fat and liver cells, where it's converted to energy or stored as fat. Many women with PCOS have insulin resistance. This means that the process of getting the sugar out of the blood and into the cells is defective – the cells are 'resistant' to insulin. The pancreas must secrete more and more insulin to get sugar out of the blood and into the cells. High levels of insulin, or *hyperinsulinaemia*, can trigger weight gain, problems with ovulation, an increased risk of diabetes, difficulty losing weight and an increased risk of heart disease by raising LDL (the unhealthy cholesterol) and triglyceride levels and decreasing HDL (the healthy cholesterol).

THYROID PROBLEMS

Your thyroid is a gland at the bottom of your neck. It weighs less than an ounce but has an enormous effect on your health. All aspects of your metabolism, from the rate at which your heart beats to how quickly you burn calories, are regulated by your thyroid hormones.

If your thyroid releases the proper amount of hormones, body systems function normally. But if your thyroid doesn't produce enough it causes *hypothyroidism* (underactive thyroid), and upsets the delicate balance of chemical reactions in your body. Symptoms include fatigue, weight gain, irregular periods and high blood pressure (sound familiar?). If you're overweight and have irregular periods and insulin resistance, it seems your risk of developing hypothyroidism is higher.

Many of the symptoms of hypothyroidism correspond with the symptoms of PCOS, and there do seem to be strong links between the two conditions. At present there just isn't enough evidence to suggest that thyroid problems may have a causal link with PCOS, but early research[10] suggests there may well be a connection of some kind.

An interesting study illustrated this by investigating the relationship between polycystic ovary syndrome, hypothyroidism and insulin-resistance and how, by submitting patients to a specific therapy for any one of these three problems, the researchers were able to obtain an improvement in the other associated conditions. [11]

This study suggests that there are several ways to improve PCOS symptoms and increase fertility. If a single therapy can be effective, a combination might be even better.

THE CORTISOL CONNECTION

There may also be a link between PCOS and the production of the stress hormone cortisol. Studies[12] have indicated that high testosterone levels associated with PCOS could be caused by a fault in the way the body produces Cortisol. This is the active form of the hormone released into the body by the adrenal gland to help it cope with stress and is turned into cortisone, the inactive form, by enzymes in the body. Researchers have found that some women with PCOS don't have these enzymes. This means their bodies cannot process cortisol properly, causing higher levels of testosterone to be produced.

This suggests that stress may play a part in the development of PCOS. If you're under stress your adrenal glands release the stress hormones –

adrenaline and cortisol, as well as testosterone – to help you cope with that stress. If there's a problem with the conversion of cortisol, you produce too much testosterone and this makes your symptoms worse and drives your body towards the classic PCOS symptoms of insulin resistance, weight gain and irregular periods. More research needs to be done, but knowing that stress may be a contributory factor can help you to take steps to 'stress-proof' your life, and you can do this with our action plan on page 266.

THE ENDOCRINE WEB

All these hormone theories – insulin, testosterone, LH, cortisol and thyroid problems – are in fact linked. This is because the endocrine (hormone) system regulating your blood sugar and insulin levels, as well as your sex hormones and stress hormones, is a sensitive web of interconnections. If one hormone is out of kilter, the others will be affected, too.

> 'We know that normal ovulation requires the perfect synchronization of hormones in the body. PCOS causes shifts in hormone levels, rendering normal ovulation unlikely. The lack of ovulation is largely to blame for the infertility aspect of PCOS, while the hormone imbalance is responsible for the associated symptoms of unwanted hair growth and acne.'[13]

Clearly in PCOS there are hormonal imbalances, but we still don't know which one is ultimately responsible for triggering the chain-reaction that causes PCOS symptoms or, in fact, if it's something external that jump-starts the imbalance.

COULD IT START IN THE WOMB?

Some researchers believe that PCOS is caused before you are born. A slight increase in testosterone levels occurs during pregnancy, especially in the first 14 weeks when the foetus' ovaries are developing. The placenta has a large amount of an enzyme called aromatase which converts testosterone into oestrogen, but there have been reports of female foetuses becoming masculinized by androgen-secreting tumours. This suggests the possibility that an excessive amount of male hormones could alter a female foetus' developing ovaries.

It's also been suggested that insulin resistance may start in the uterus. If the mother is nutrient deficient, it's possible that she sends a signal to her foetus that starvation is a possibility. The foetus, therefore, becomes insulin resistant as in times of famine, because the fat storage that this encourages has certain advantages. So far, studies[14] haven't confirmed this hypothesis, but if it were true then low-weight or small babies would have a higher risk of PCOS, when in fact the opposite is true: research[15] has shown that babies who are overweight and overdue have a higher risk of developing PCOS later in life.

IS YOUR WEIGHT TO BLAME?

Being overweight increases insulin levels dramatically and makes PCOS symptoms worse. Studies[16] have shown that losing weight can not only reduce the symptoms of PCOS but can also help normalize ovulation, boost fertility and resolve hormonal problems.

Weight loss is so beneficial because it results in lower insulin levels, which in turn can reduce testosterone levels. Trouble is, as you'll see in Part 2, if you've got PCOS you're far more likely to have difficulty losing weight.

But does weight gain *cause* PCOS? Even though a woman with PCO who puts a lot of weight on might start to get PCOS symptoms, most experts believe that weight gain is a symptom, not a cause, of the syndrome, because research[17] shows that slim women can and do report PCOS symptoms too.

DIET AND LIFESTYLE TRIGGERS?

Fertility studies indicate that both eating disorders and poor diets (e.g. diets high in fat, sugar and carbohydrate and low in nutrients) can and do affect the function of the ovaries. This is because a poor diet triggers the release of too much insulin, increasing the risk of an overproduction of testosterone and PCOS. And it's been suggested[18] that nearly two-thirds of women with bulimia may have PCOS.

So does a poor diet cause PCOS, or does PCOS trigger fad dieting because of the need to control weight gain, or even bingeing and purging due to sugar cravings set off by insulin resistance? The jury's still out, though many women with PCOS believe the link is there.

'I know science has yet to prove it, but I certainly believe my own PCOS was made a lot worse by my bingeing and starving cycle. As a teenager I was desperate not to be so dumpy and starved myself on stupid diets, but my spots, my weight and my irregular periods just got worse and worse.'
Emma, 32

Some researchers[19] believe that when PCOS runs in families it isn't because of a genetic reason; rather other factors common in families – typically a poor diet and lack of exercise leading to overproduction of insulin. Again, all this has yet to be proved conclusively, but what we do know for sure is that one of the best ways to manage PCOS is to clean up your act when it comes to diet and lifestyle. Part 2 will give you plenty of advice on how to do just that.

'For centuries, experts in the studies of philosophy, science and medicine have pondered the question of how much of who we are is inherited and how much in due to environment. There is no medical issue that begs the answer for this question more than does PCOS.'[20]

HORMONE DISRUPTERS

Xenoestrogens or endocrine-disrupting chemicals (EDCs) are widely recognized to be highly toxic in the smallest doses. Despite this, they exist throughout our environment, from pesticide residues on food to pollution in our air and water to medications and the high-sugar, preserved and processed fast foods in our diet.

EDCs are characterized as 'hormone disrupters' because they have a molecular structure similar to the hormone oestrogen and can interfere with the natural process of your hormones. They trick your body into a condition known as oestrogen excess or oestrogen dominance, and the resulting hormonal imbalance can trigger a wide variety of PCOS symptoms, from irregular periods and acne to dry hair and weight gain.

'You hear so much about pollution reducing men's sperm counts, but no-one talks about how the same pollution affects women. I want to know more!'

Aileen, 37

Research[21] about how EDCs affect or trigger PCOS is still in its infancy, but we know enough to suggest that exposure to hormone-disrupting toxins could be a contributory factor – that's why you'll find a chapter in Part 2 devoted to this important issue.

IS IT ALL IN THE MIND?

Does PCOS have something to do with your mental or emotional state? Some researchers believe that it might, in two ways: first, studies[22] show it may be caused or triggered by epilepsy or at least one of the medications routinely used (depakote or valproate) to treat epileptic seizures. Second, other studies[23] indicate that PCOS may worsen mood and anxiety symptoms.

This is a controversial area of research with potentially huge consequences for the recognition and treatment of PCOS as not just a hormonal disorder but also a mood disorder.

If you've got PCOS you probably don't need a study to tell you that the symptoms can turn your mood black and crank up your anxiety levels from time to time – that's why Part 3 of this book is packed with advice on stress-reduction and getting yourself in the right frame of mind to take charge of your mood and your symptoms.

BETA CELL FUNCTION

Insulin is produced by the beta cells of the pancreas; researchers are currently investigating whether women with PCOS have a beta-cell function that is more responsive to insulin resistance than women without PCOS. Early studies[24] indicate that this may indeed be the case. Further research in this field could well lead to discoveries of new therapies and better diagnoses for women with PCOS and insulin resistance.

METABOLIC SYNDROME (SYNDROME X)

Metabolic Syndrome or Syndrome X is a term used to describe a set of risk factors that increase the risk of heart attack by 4 to 20 times. These factors include insulin resistance, weight gain around the tummy, high levels of blood fats and high blood pressure. It's thought to be caused by the body's inability to process a diet high in sugary foods and refined carbohydrates. These refined carbohydrates not only drive the body to insulin resistance but also fail to supply the many nutrients the body needs for hormones to function at optimum levels.

Many women with PCOS have symptoms of Syndrome X – and as it seems possible that men could get PCOS too (see page 13) – could PCOS simply be a female version of symptoms that are triggered by Metabolic Syndrome? Could Syndrome X be the cardiologist's view of what a gynaecologist would call PCOS? Much more research[25] needs to be done.

HOW DO THESE THEORIES HELP ME?

In the end, the most important thing about all the research into PCOS is that it will help scientists, the medical community, natural health practitioners and women who have PCOS to work out the best ways of dealing with it. But the underlying results of most research so far has one thing in common – the best thing any woman with PCOS can do for herself is to take charge of her environment – diet, lifestyle, emotional health – in order to redress the hormonal imbalances within her endocrine system and restore better health. That's why Parts 2 and 3 of this book are packed with practical information on how to get the help that works best for you and your specific symptoms. And the best thing about these self-help measures is that you can use them with whatever type of medication you decide to take.

Chapter 5 will take a look at what the medical community can offer, but before we launch into medication let's complete this preliminary overview of PCOS by taking a look at how it affects your hormonal life stages from puberty to the menopause and beyond.

CHAPTER 3
PCOS AND YOUR LIFE STAGES – FROM PUBERTY TO MENOPAUSE

It's clear that there can be different stages of PCOS throughout your life. Studies[1] show, for instance, that younger women tend to have substantial difficulties with their periods, whereas older women[2] tend to have other problems such as diabetes and hypertension (high blood pressure).

PCOS symptoms often appear first during puberty, though – as mentioned in Chapter 2 – recent research suggests that PCOS may begin even earlier. According to lead author David Abbott, Ph.D., of the Wisconsin National Primate Center at the University of Wisconsin-Madison,[3] PCOS develops in the first and second trimesters of pregnancy when excess androgens are present.

But for now, here's what we know about how PCOS affects your hormonal life stages, from puberty to menopause and beyond.

PUBERTY AND PCOS

Puberty is the beginning of a physical transformation towards fertility, which usually takes about four years to complete. Body shape, hormone levels and behaviour all begin to change in response to hormonal instructions. Breasts develop, pubic hair grows, bones strengthen and height and weight increase.

In women without PCOS, before the onset of puberty, the pituitary gland prompts the ovaries and adrenal glands to start producing larger amounts of the sex hormones oestrogen and androgen.

Oestrogens, often known as the 'female' hormones, control breast development and changes in the vagina and its excretions. Before the first menstrual period (called *menarche*), levels of oestrogen in the bloodstream begin to fluctuate widely. The womb lining (endometrium) is affected by these hormonal changes until a point is reached when it starts to grow.

Meanwhile androgens, often known as the 'male' hormones, control the growth of pubic hair under the arms and in the pubic area, stimulate growth and weight gain and speed up the maturation of the bones and an increase in muscle mass. But androgens mostly come to a teenage girl's attention when they cause that common and unwanted effect of puberty – acne.

These physical changes may also be accompanied by emotional conflicts, some of which are hormonally triggered. Sudden, unpredictable mood swings in adolescents can be due to the surges in these hormones (think about any PMS or PCOS mood swings you get and it might take you back to your teens).

FIRST OVULATION

The first ovulation doesn't occur until around six to nine months after a girl's first period.

The mechanisms for initiating menstruation are present in a child's brain and pituitary gland from birth, but something keeps them turned off until puberty. Many scientists believe this is weight, with a body-fat ratio of around 25 per cent being the trigger. It's thought that the hormone leptin, produced by fat cells, must achieve a certain level in the blood in order for menstruation to occur, and that this level must be sustained for the menstrual cycle to be regular.

As body weight during puberty increases it's thought that the hypothalamus triggers the release of gonadotrophin-releasing hormone (GnRH). It's thought that the body fat ratio triggers the onset of menstruation, some time between the ages of 11 and 18.

GnRH then stimulates the pituitary to release follicle-stimulating hormone (FSH) and luteinizing hormone (LH). As we've seen in Chapter 1, in sexually mature females FSH and LH act on the follicle to stimulate it to release oestrogens and trigger the maturing of the egg and its release (ovulation) in the middle of the cycle. Later, LH stimulates the empty follicle to develop into the corpus luteum, which secretes progesterone during the latter part of the menstrual cycle to prepare the body for a possible pregnancy.

Somehow the brain senses the body mass or fat mass, and only lets puberty start when a certain weight is reached, typically around 7 stone (100 lb), although this can vary considerably. This would explain why petite girls often get their periods later than heavier or taller ones. It would also explain why some women stop getting periods when they lose too much weight (think of gymnasts, or women with anorexia or even athletes in hard training). Although this theory has its problems, as some very thin women do menstruate, it does make sense that pregnancy shouldn't occur until a body has enough fat stores to see it through successfully.

Research[4] indicates that a healthy diet with a balance of fats, proteins and carbohydrates is important for the onset and continuation of menstruation, whether a woman has PCOS or not. In the 1830s women typically began menstruation at the age of 17, while today the average age is 13. This change is thought to be linked to improved nutrition, but some argue that it's due to rising obesity levels and exposure to hormones in the environment and to food additives.

Once menstruation has started, a continual release of the hormone GnRH is essential to keep periods regular. Stress and sudden body weight changes can upset the release of this hormone and cause irregular or absent periods. Again, perhaps this is the body's way of ensuring that pregnancy only occurs when a woman's mind and body are ready to support it.

HOW PCOS AFFECTS PUBERTY

In general, many girls with PCOS have a puberty that is normal in every respect except when it comes to periods. Breast and hair development are normal, as is the increase in weight and height, but a normal menstrual cycle isn't established. Periods are either absent or irregular. Apart from the irregular periods, other typical symptoms of PCOS may not be present.

Some other research[5] has suggested that girls with premature puberty who develop pubic hair early (say before the age of 8) have many of the signs and symptoms of PCOS. Throughout puberty these girls produces excess testosterone and have irregular periods. So, premature puberty could be an early sign of PCOS.

Some adolescent girls experience many of the same symptoms as adults – especially irregular or absent periods, unwanted hair, weight gain and acne. In rare cases these symptoms can occur very rapidly. A young girl may gain 30 or so pounds in a few months, even though her diet has not changed, or she might notice more and more dark hair on her chin and upper lip.

▷ IF YOU SUSPECT YOUR DAUGHTER MAY HAVE PCOS

Adolescence is a tough time for a girl regardless of whether she has PCOS or not. But for girls with PCOS, it can be even tougher. They can often feel isolated and confused. At an age when appearance seems to be everything, girls with PCOS lose a great deal of self-confidence when their symptoms start appearing. This is made worse because many girls feel they haven't got anyone to talk or feel too embarrassed to seek help.

If you suspect your daughter might have PCOS, either because her symptoms are physically obvious or because you know her cycle is irregular, it's very important that you find a doctor who knows about PCOS and can diagnose it.

Puberty may seem chaotic but it does follow an orderly process, and if events fall out of line questions should be asked. If there's early hair growth, or no period 12 months after breast and pubic hair development, or excessive acne or abnormal hair growth, do make sure you seek help and advice. You should also consult your daughter's doctor if six months after they start her periods are very frequent, excessive or far apart.

Do be aware that, even today with increased awareness of PCOS, some doctors pass off early signs as 'typical' teenage symptoms – hair growth, acne, mood swings are common to many teenagers, after all. If you're concerned, seek a second or a third opinion – when a health-care provider takes the time to explain what PCOS is and offers treatment options, a young woman may feel relieved that at last there's an explanation and treatment for her problems. And an early start with control measures can make a real difference to health, self-image and quality of life.

Many girls with PCOS tell us that talking with a counsellor about their concerns can be very helpful, as can joining a support group for girls who have PCOS. (See our recommended websites for great online links.)

Generally the tests for PCOS in teens are the same as those for women, as are the treatment options offered, such as the contraceptive pill and metformin. The lifestyle and self-help advice given in Part 2 of this book can be broadly applied to teens as well.

PCOS AND FERTILITY

Many women with PCOS are diagnosed in their twenties and thirties, but some aren't diagnosed until they are in their forties. This is because it's during this time a woman is most likely to want to conceive, and many women with PCOS aren't diagnosed until they have trouble getting pregnant. (This is a concern, as PCOS is far more than a fertility issue and has long-term health effects.)

You'll find plenty of information about boosting fertility in Part 2.

PCOS AND PREGNANCY

Despite fertility problems, 70 per cent of women with PCOS do conceive naturally. It might be logical to assume that PCOS is 'cured' or goes away when you get pregnant – after all, you've ovulated – but unfortunately this isn't the case. 'Although some women with PCOS find that their post pregnancy cycles get more regular, there isn't any evidence to suggest that pregnancy cures PCOS,' says PCOS expert Adam Balen. 'What we do know, though, is that research does seem to indicate that a PCOS pregnancy is at greater risk.' While it may seem scary to read about the risks, knowing about them means you can deal with them in a proactive and positive way.

Research[6] suggests that women with PCOS are more likely to miscarry, possibly due to excess weight, which is itself associated with an increased risk of miscarriage. It could also be due to the higher LH concentrations in PCOS, which could damage egg quality.

PCOS may also increase the risk of gestational diabetes[7] (diabetes that occurs during pregnancy) due to weight issues and/or insulin resistance, and this ups the risk of hypertension and the need for a Caesarean section during labour.

Pregnant women with PCOS who are insulin resistant are also at an increased risk of hypertension or high blood pressure.[8] Pregnancy-induced hypertension carries with it the risk of growth retardation in the baby and damage to the nervous system and kidneys in the mother.

We know this all sounds alarming, but do remember that every pregnancy carries risks, whether you have PCOS or not. And if your doctor is aware, and works with you to monitor your pregnancy closely, you should pick up any early warning signs.

PERIMENOPAUSE AND THE MENOPAUSE

In the same way as a car can't go from 60 mph to standstill without slowing down, your ovaries also need time to slow down before they stop completely at the onset of the menopause. Perimenopause is the period of gradual physical and biochemical change that leads to the menopause, when your ovaries' production of oestrogen slows down, causing irregular periods. Generally changes such as shorter or longer periods, heavier or lighter bleeding and varying lengths of time between periods may be an indication of perimenopause, which usually lasts around two to five years, before the menopause itself – your last period. The average age for the onset of perimenopause is 47, though this varies.

Typical symptoms of perimenopause include fatigue, mood swings, hot flushes, vaginal dryness, loss of libido, memory loss, night sweats and irregular periods.

The average age of the menopause for women in Western nations is 51, though some may experience it as early as their thirties or as late as their sixties due to hereditary influences or even illness. You're classified as post-menopausal when you haven't had a period for 12 months.

PCOS AND THE PERIMENOPAUSE

Perimenopause can often go unnoticed in women with PCOS, as they are used to having irregular periods. Some women with PCOS say that, instead of their cycles becoming more irregular, they actually become more regular. A possible explanation for this is that the hormonal swings and high oestrogen and androgen levels associated with PCOS may lessen as a woman nears the menopause, when oestrogen and androgen levels naturally lower.

Many women with PCOS assume that because they've always had irregular periods they won't go through the menopause. This isn't the case. Whether you have PCOS or not, the menopause causes a significant decrease in oestrogen and this can increase the risk of heart disease, osteoporosis and cancer, so you do need to manage it.

Many of the symptoms of the menopause are related to this drop in oestrogen, and you can still expect these changes if you've got PCOS.

According to research, the high levels of androgen in PCOS may fall during the menopause, sometimes to normal levels, although they usually remain higher than for women who don't have PCOS. But many androgen-related problems, such as increased hair growth (hirsutism) and acne, continue (although they rarely get worse).

The risk of heart disease increases for all women after the menopause, but women with PCOS are at even higher risk due to raised androgen levels, unhealthy changes to blood fats and obesity. In addition, 40 per cent of women with PCOS develop Type 2 diabetes by the age of 40, which further increases the risk of heart disease.

For this reason you should make sure your doctor regularly checks your blood fat levels and blood pressure.

'I always thought menopause would be the end of it all. What a shocker to find out that this is a myth!'

Linda, 49

HRT OR NOT HRT?

In the past, HRT (hormone replacement therapy) has been widely used to help women going through the menopause and post-menopause. Some doctors even prescribe it for perimenopause if hot flushes are a problem. What research there is suggests that taking HRT can bring about the same benefits for women with PCOS as it does for women without PCOS. But because of the increased risk of cancer of the endometrium (womb), women with PCOS should use a type of HRT that includes progesterone to induce periods. Androgenic progesterones, such as levonorgesterel, should be avoided.

Also bear in mind that recent research on the effects of HRT (since 2003) has led doctors to question whether any possible long-term benefits are worth the risks associated with the treatment, such as an increased risk of breast cancer and heart disease if you take it for more than five years. You should be aware of these risks and how they might compare with the possible benefits when deciding what you want to do.

If you're considering hormone replacement therapy, do make sure your doctor is familiar with PCOS and can help you select a treatment plan that will take into consideration the specific problems associated with PCOS.

You may of course decide not to go down the HRT route, and protect yourself with diet and lifestyle changes instead. If this is the case, it's still important that you keep in close touch with your doctor to make sure you're protected against the long-term health risks associated with PCOS.

'My mother died of breast cancer at 56, so there was absolutely no way I was going to go on HRT.'
Maureen, 57

AFTER THE MENOPAUSE

Because we now have longer life spans and often live well into our eighties, modern women are usually post-menopausal for a third of their lives.

So does PCOS fade away after the menopause? 'This is probably the most asked question by women over age 40 with PCOS,' says PCOS expert Samuel Thatcher, 'The answer to which is, No!'

This was shown in a study[9] from Kaplan Medical Centre in Israel, which evaluated 104 post-menopausal women by physical examination, detailed questionnaire and laboratory measurements of glucose, blood fats and sex-hormone levels. Seven (6.7 per cent) of the women were diagnosed with PCOS. As compared to women without PCOS, central obesity (fat around the stomach) was more common in the PCOS group, 4 out of 7 had Type 2 diabetes compared to 8 out of 97 in the non-PCOS group, and 6 out of 7 (versus 31 out of 97) had elevated blood fats (triglycerides, cholesterol) characteristic of the Metabolic Syndrome (Syndrome X). PCOS appears to be fairly common in post-menopausal women, and is a marker for a metabolic profile associated with a high risk of cardiovascular diseases.

'I really noticed "middle-aged spread" as I put weight on my tummy. But then so did my friends without PCOS when they went through menopause.'
Jan, 56

To recap: We know that women with PCOS are already at an increased risk of developing diabetes, heart disease and endometrial cancer. Because such risks only increase with age, treating PCOS both during and after the menopause is essential.

SAVING THE BEST TILL LAST

From our many chats with women with PCOS it's very clear that this post-menopause stage in life offers a wonderful and liberating opportunity to understand ourselves, our sexuality and what we have to contribute to the world. In the words of Sally, age 52:

'I think there are many things to love about being post-menopausal. PCOS is still there but I'm finding it's easier to manage. There's a light at the end of the tunnel of heavy bleeding, no bleeding, nightmare PMS and hot flushes. No more worry about pregnancy. Most women find their voice and have no qualms about raising it. This doesn't happen overnight, of course, and for many women it takes time to stop feeling bad about speaking up – but they realize they've nothing to lose and a lot to gain!

'Many women find another vocation of sorts for their "second act". With children out of the house or getting older, they can spend time on themselves, go back to school and take a class in a subject they have always dreamt about. Some pick up a paint brush for the first time, try a musical instrument or write a best-seller. Others have relationships, get married for the first time or again, start a business or travel the world. Of course these aren't snap decisions and take months if not years of meditation and consultation with family and friends. But the possibilities are endless.'

CHAPTER 4
WHAT AM I DEALING WITH?

Below you'll find a list of the key short- and long-term symptoms that women with PCOS are *likely* to have. We stress *likely*, as your symptoms will be unique to you and different from those of another woman with the syndrome. There's a wide menu of PCOS symptoms out there, and you can get any combination to any degree of severity, which is why it's important to find the solutions that work for you.

The most important thing to note is that PCOS is a combination of day-to-day symptoms and longer-term health effects. Even if your day-to-day symptoms aren't bothering you so much, don't ignore the self-help plans that come later in the book – the long-term health risks of PCOS mean you need to take action *now*.

'The thing that got me started on a self-help plan was worrying about diabetes, but actually I lost some weight and got less spotty just from eating better and getting fitter, and I feel great!'

Amy-Jay, 29

EARLY SIGNS

Many symptoms of polycystic ovary syndrome (PCOS) start gradually, and you may think they're related to some other medical problem.

IRREGULAR PERIODS

Nine or fewer menstrual cycles per year, or no menstrual cycles at all, may be one of the most common signs of PCOS. When periods *do* occur, they may be heavier, longer and more painful than normal. These conditions are caused by a hormone imbalance. Almost 50 per cent of women with PCOS don't ovulate every month.

EXCESS HAIR

Sometimes called 'hirsutism', this can be a difficult symptom if you have it. For most women with PCOS, hair in the moustache and beard areas becomes heavier and darker. Masculine hair on the arms and legs, and excess hair in the pubic region, abdomen, chest or back, or on your thumbs or toes, is also possible. This symptom is caused by high levels of male hormones (androgens), as are thinning hair and acne. Up to 70 per cent of women with PCOS complain of excess hair growth.

'One of the things that bugs me most is the hairs around my nipples.'
Harriet, 42

SKIN PROBLEMS

Skin problems such as acne, oily skin or dandruff can also crop up, due to excess testosterone. The acne is usually found around the face (especially along the jaw line), chest and back. Also, dark skin patches (*acanthosis nigricans*) on the neck, groin, underarms, or in skin folds, or skin tags (*acrochordons*) in the armpits or neck area can also bother women with PCOS. These are related to insulin resistance and diabetes.

'I can't believe I still have spots at the age of 30!'
Karen

GRADUALLY DEVELOPING SYMPTOMS

MOOD SWINGS

These may be caused by the emotional problems or body image insecurities related to, and triggered by the physical symptoms of PCOS, but they can also be a result of hormonal imbalance – if you've ever experienced PMS you'll know how hormones can affect your feelings.

WEIGHT GAIN

'Apple-shape' weight gain, or upper-body obesity (more abdominal fat than hip fat) is also known as android obesity and is associated with increased testosterone levels. Many women with PCOS gain weight around their middle, and this type of weight gain can increase your risk of insulin resistance and diabetes.

Yes, it's official. If you've got PCOS you're not only more likely to be overweight but more likely to find it hard to lose weight. Research[1] shows that obesity is four times more likely in women with PCOS and irregular periods than those without. And the tendency[2] is to put on weight around the waist rather than the hips. Researchers think they've discovered the reason for this. Studies[3] show that women with PCOS actually store fat more efficiently and burn calories more slowly than women without PCOS, even when they are on a diet.

In Part 2 we'll explain in more detail what research has uncovered and, more importantly what you can do to kick-start weight loss, but for now if you're struggling with your weight just bear in mind that you're not alone and there are things you can do about it. If you're struggling, we have an action plan in Chapter 11.

FERTILITY PROBLEMS

If you don't have regular menstrual cycles, you may have problems getting pregnant. This isn't the same as infertility, though – with help, most women with PCOS can get pregnant.

INSULIN RESISTANCE

For women with PCOS, insulin resistance increases the risk of developing diabetes. You may also develop diabetes at a younger age because of PCOS. About 30 per cent of women with PCOS have impaired glucose functioning, and 7 to 10 per cent have Type 2 diabetes. Some symptoms associated with insulin resistance include skin changes, such as skin tags or dark skin patches and upper-body weight gain.

MALE PATTERN BALDNESS

Just as heavier hair growth on your face and body is possible, thinning hair (alopecia) is also a symptom of PCOS. This is caused by higher levels of androgens.

SLEEP APNOEA

This has been reported to occur in up to 30 per cent of women with PCOS who are overweight. It's a disorder characterized by excessive snoring at night with brief spells where breathing stops completely. Patients with this problem experience fatigue and daytime sleepiness. It can be diagnosed by a sleep study, and there are a variety of treatments available.

THE LONG-TERM HEALTH RISKS

Some conditions related to PCOS may not be obvious but are potentially dangerous. The long-term health risks[4] include:

- Diabetes – about 30 per cent of women with PCOS have a problem processing blood sugar (glucose intolerance). This is a major risk factor for adult-onset diabetes.
- High blood pressure – if you've got PCOS, research[5] shows that your risk of hypertension is higher than normal. This is because weight gain, high cholesterol levels and insulin resistance are known risk factors for high blood pressure.

- Heart and blood vessel disease – people with high insulin levels, as in PCOS, often have low levels of so-called good cholesterol (HDL cholesterol) and high levels of other fats, including triglycerides. These factors are known to increase the risk of heart attack or stroke later in life.

- Uterine cancer – if you don't have regular periods, the lining of the uterus may not shed as often as it should, and instead build up and grow thicker, increasing the risk of cancer of the uterus. If PCOS goes untreated, this may increase the risk of cancer of the uterus.

There are some other conditions that women and/or PCOS experts suspect may be linked to PCOS, though research has yet to confirm this:

- Breast cancer – some studies have suggested that women with PCOS have an increased risk due to the obesity link and the hormonal fluctuations that can lead to an excess of oestrogen in the body and irregular periods. Other studies,[6] however, haven't found this link.

- Eating disorders – a recent study suggested that PCOS doesn't cause eating disorders, but as weight-management problems are a common symptom of PCOS it's hardly surprising that research[7] suggests that as many as 60 per cent of women with PCOS may have eating disorders, such as bulimia.

- Osteoporosis (brittle bones) – women with PCOS and unhealthy eating patterns such as bulimia just aren't giving their bones the nutrients they need to stay healthy and strong.

- Thyroid imbalance – since the hormonal systems in your body are all interconnected, it's logical to assume that the hormonal havoc PCOS causes could trigger an imbalance in thyroid hormone production.

- Chronic Pelvic Pain – some women with PCOS suffer from chronic pelvic pain. Although no research has been done it's not difficult to see why women with PCOS think there may be a link with their PCOS.

- Digestive complaints – many women with PCOS complain of digestive problems, in particular constipation and Irritable Bowel Syndrome. So far research has not discovered why this is the case, but it may have something to do with the slightly lowered metabolic rate associated with PCOS, which would make your digestive system a bit slower.

- Lowered immunity – many women with PCOS say they get ill more than women without PCOS. There could be an explanation for this. Research[8] has suggested a link between lowered immunity and menstrual irregularity. It seems the high levels of testosterone associated with PCOS cause a fault in the way the body processes the stress hormone cortisol, so the body's ability to deal with stress is weakened. And people under stress are more likely to get ill.

- Fatigue – although fatigue and lack of energy aren't officially recognized as symptoms of PCOS, the hormonal fluctuations and blood sugar issues suggest energy levels could be an issue.

- Endometriosis – it's not uncommon to see both PCOS and endometriosis in the same woman. Some experts believe the two conditions are not only similar but may be linked in some way.

- Ovarian cancer – a 1996 study reported an increased risk of ovarian cancer among women with PCOS, but more recent research suggests that the link is by no means established.

- Depression – some experts believe that depression, in particular bi-polar disorder, is more common in women with PCOS, but is there a direct biological cause or is it because dealing with PCOS can just really get you down?

- Asthma – could the excess oestrogen associated with PCOS worsen asthma? Research[9] indicates that women with irregular periods have higher rates of asthma and allergy than women with regular periods. Metabolic problems, such as insulin resistance, have been suggested as an underlying cause for both.
- Fibroids – there is no doubt that fibroids are related to oestrogen levels. Could they also be related to PCOS?

CHAPTER 5
HOW CAN MY DOCTOR HELP?

Your doctor is most likely to suggest a combination of medication and lifestyle modifications to help you control the signs and symptoms of PCOS. Medical and surgical treatment can also help you if you're having trouble conceiving.

Do bear in mind that your treatment will be unique to you and will depend upon your individual symptoms. If you do decide to take medication we would strongly urge you to take an active role in your medical care by learning as much as you can about the condition and by working with your doctor to develop the best treatment plan for *you*.

TREATING IRREGULAR PERIODS

If you have irregular periods, your doctor is most likely to prescribe you oral contraceptives. In addition to protecting the uterine lining by inducing a monthly bleed, some brands of contraceptive pill can control excess face and body hair. And, of course, you get the contraceptive benefit.

Before prescribing oral contraceptives, your doctor will perform an examination or a blood test to be certain that you aren't pregnant. If you haven't had a period for six weeks or longer, your doctor may also first prescribe medroxyprogesterone acetate or a progestin (Provera) to induce a menstrual period. A progestin is a medication that mimics the action of progesterone. This will cause a period in almost all women with PCOS, but it doesn't help with the cosmetic concerns (excess hair or acne) and doesn't provide contraception.

A modest amount of weight loss can also restore normal periods in some women. For example, many overweight women with PCOS who lose 5 to 10 per cent of their body weight notice that their periods become more regular.

The final treatment for irregular menstrual periods is the use of insulin-lowering agents (see page 55).

POSSIBLE SIDE-EFFECTS

Some women who take oral contraceptives (not just those with PCOS) may notice amenorrhoea (lack of menstrual periods) or breakthrough bleeding (bleeding that occurs at the wrong time of the month). Often this breakthrough bleeding settles down after a few menstrual cycles, but if it happens your doctor may order an ultrasound scan of the uterus to check your endometrium (uterine lining).

If ultrasound shows that the endometrium is very thin, and if you don't mind having no periods, your doctor may simply recommend continuing with oral contraceptives. If you prefer having menstrual periods, the type and dosage of contraceptives can be changed.

If the ultrasound shows that the endometrium is thick, your doctor will often prescribe a different type and dosage of oral contraceptives to trigger a period.

Many women worry that they will gain weight on the Pill. In the early days of the Pill this was a real problem; however, with the low-oestrogen pills now used, weight gain is very unusual. Nausea and bloating are potential side-effects, but these symptoms almost always go away after two or three months of taking the Pill.

Some women also say that the Pill increases their appetite. The British Medical Association's *Official Guide to Medicines and Drugs*,[1] does list weight gain as a possible side-effect. It goes on to say that 'Oestrogen may also trigger the onset of diabetes mellitus in susceptible people, or aggravate blood sugar control in diabetic women.' This isn't usually a concern, but if you have PCOS you are at an increased risk of obesity and insulin resistance already, so you need to discuss this carefully with your doctor.

In addition, blood clots can occur, although this is a rare complication in healthy women. The risk of a healthy woman developing blood clots with the contraceptive pill is estimated at just 1 in 30,000.

While the Pill is thought to be very safe and effective, it's important that we point out that it might lower your libido and can occasionally raise blood pressure, as well as cholesterol, blood sugar, and insulin levels.[2] A preliminary study reported in the January 2006 *Journal of Sexual Medicine* claims that taking the contraceptive pill may lead to long-term loss of libido. A US–Canadian study[3] has also found that even low-dose oral contraceptives appear to increase women's risk of a heart attack or stroke. Dr John Nestler and Dr Paulina Essah of Virginia Commonwealth University, and Dr Jean-Patrice Baillargeon of the Université de Sherbrooke, analysed the results of several studies published between 1980 and 2002. They determined that women using low-dose contraceptives have approximately twice the risk of stroke or heart disease.

Women with polycystic ovary syndrome already have an increased risk of cardiovascular disease, Dr Nestler said, and are at an even greater risk if they are treated with low-dose contraceptives. He suggested that doctors consider alternatives. Long-term use of oral contraceptives may also increase this risk, Nestler said. But he said that for most women the risk is still very low.

This study reinforces why we emphasize the importance of natural approaches for treating PCOS, such as a healthy diet, regular exercise, stress management and selected nutritional supplements and herbs. Hormone contraception is effective in preventing pregnancy, but should be chosen with a full understanding of the health risks involved. Always consider alternatives including barrier methods (diaphragm, cervical cap, IUD, condoms), which have the added benefit of protecting you against sexually-transmitted diseases (STDs).

There are also health risks associated with being on the Pill if you're overweight. Synthetic oestrogens in the Pill can increase the body's drive towards insulin resistance, a precursor to diabetes. There's also the increased risk of high blood pressure. So, for women with PCOS who have weight problems being on the Pill isn't a good idea unless you're following a healthy eating, healthy living plan and having regular check-ups for blood pressure, blood sugar and blood cholesterol levels.

Finally, it's important to stress that the pill is *not* a miracle cure, because although it results in monthly menstrual periods, this doesn't mean your PCOS is 'cured'. But if it's the right option for you, having a healthy lifestyle is the key.

Some studies[4] also suggest that the Pill may actually leach valuable nutrients as well as alter your vitamin and mineral levels. Research indicates that the Pill lowers levels of B vitamins, folic acid, vitamin C and vitamin E. Levels of vitamin A and iron may also increase, as do levels of copper – which isn't a good thing because copper levels that are higher than normal can increase the risk of high blood pressure. Zinc is perhaps the most important mineral that can be affected by the Pill. The Pill is thought to change a woman's capacity to absorb zinc, and you need sufficient levels of zinc to maintain a healthy reproductive system and hormonal balance.

If you're on the Pill, on top of your healthy diet (which we'll outline in Part 2) it might be a good idea to supplement extra vitamin B complex to help your liver break down synthetic hormones effectively. You might also consider taking a zinc supplement.

We also know that the Pill can lower levels of good cholesterol (HDL) and increase levels of bad cholesterol (LDL), so you need to eat foods that promote good cholesterol to reduce your risk of heart disease. The Pill can also kill off friendly bacteria in your gut, which can lead to digestive problems. Live yoghurt which contains natural probiotics should be on your daily menu. If you're dairy intolerant, you can buy fruit-based drinks with live bacterial cultures from health food stores.

WHICH PILL IS BEST FOR PCOS?

Oral contraceptives come in two types — ones containing both oestrogen and progesterone, and ones that contain only progesterone. The combined (oestrogen and progesterone) contraceptive is the most widely prescribed because it's the most reliable. There are many different products available and they are divided into three groups depending on their oestrogen content:

1. Low-dose brands such as Minulet, Ovran, Femodene, Loestrin and Ovranette
2. Medium-dose brands such as Brevinor, Cilest, Norimin and Ovysmen
3. High-dose brands such as Norinly-l, Ortho Novin 1/50 and Ovran.

There are also pills that come in two or three groups, or phases, each phase containing a different proportion of oestrogen and progesterone, such as Triadene, TriMinulet, TriNordial and TriNovum. (Please note brand names may differ outside the UK.)

Progesterone-only pills are slightly less reliable and must be taken at exactly the same time each day. UK brand names include Femulen, Micoval, Norgeston and Noriday.

You might think that progesterone-only pills are the best choice if you've got PCOS, but some women have found that progesterone-only pills or pills with low doses of oestrogen don't properly suppress their PCOS symptoms, or even make them worse. One study[5] found that the contraceptives with the greatest risk of triggering diabetes were progestin-only pills (progestin is a synthetic form of progesterone). However, a study from Harvard Medical School placed the blame for this increased risk not on the Pill but on excess weight. Of all the contraceptives studied, the combination pill containing norethindrome appeared to be the safest and did not increase the risk of diabetes.

According to Dr Helen Mason, senior lecturer in Reproductive Endocrinology at St George's Hospital Medical School, London, certain brands may make androgenic effects (hair growth or loss and other 'masculinizing' symptoms) worse:

'Norethisterone found in Brevinor, Loestrin, Trinovum, is the most androgenic and should be avoided. The next most androgenic is levonorgestrel found in logynon, Microgynon, Ovran and then Desogestrel found in Marvelon. It seems that cyproterene acetate found in Dianette is the least androgenic and as a result is commonly prescribed for hirsutism, Dianette is probably your best choice.'

Cilest is another brand to choose if excess body hair is a problem. If you're prone to acne you need to go for contraceptive pills with the new progesterones such as Minulet, Femodene, Ovysmen, Brevinor or Yasmin.

Weight gain tends to be more common with the higher-dose pills – which are now, thankfully, almost a thing of the past. Switching to lower-dose pills may help, but bear in mind that even lower-dose oestrogen pills can cause water retention, and that progesterone can still increase your appetite. If weight gain is a concern, go for the pills with the newest progesterones, such as Femodene, to reduce the risk, but always check with your doctor that it's the right pill for you and your symptoms. If you're on a low-dose pill there's no reason why, with careful attention to your diet and regular exercise, you shouldn't be able to manage your weight.

It's hard to say how long you should stay on the Pill, as every woman is different. You need to discuss this carefully with your doctor. The best advice is to monitor your health and your symptoms carefully. If you think the Pill is making things worse, tell your doctor. You may also find that after taking one brand of pill for several years your symptoms seem to be returning, perhaps as a result of increased insulin resistance. If you think your pill is triggering weight gain and your symptoms, ask your doctor for advice.

EXCESS HAIR AND ACNE TREATMENTS

Oral contraceptives such as Dianette and Yasmin decrease your body's production of androgens, as do anti-androgen drugs such as spironolactone. Both treatments can lessen and slow hair growth. Oral contraceptives and anti-androgens can also reduce acne in women with PCOS, although some women may also need topical and/or oral antibiotics. Persistent cases of acne may require consultation with a dermatologist.

Excess hair can be removed with local measures such as shaving, use of depilatories, electrolysis and laser therapy. Many women worry that these local measures make hair grow faster, but this isn't true.

Electrolysis is a permanent form of hair removal but it has several drawbacks. First, there are no standardized licensing guidelines for electrolysis, so finding an experienced, effective technician is difficult. Second, this method requires repeated treatments for up to 12 or 18 months. Finally, side-effects can include pain, infection, keloid (scar) formation (for people who are susceptible), hyperpigmentation (darker patches of skin), or hypopigmentation (lighter patches of skin).

Studies[6] show that laser treatment can be effective, though it can be expensive.

Vaniqa is a prescription-only topical cream which many women have found to be particularly effective and suitable for unwanted hair growth associated with PCOS.

Vaniqa is applied twice a day to areas of unwanted facial hair. Noticeable results are usually observed after 4–8 weeks, but you need to keep using the cream or the hair will grow back. A common side-effect is acne, unfortunately, but many women have found it helpful nevertheless. Vaniqa is licensed in the US, and some UK doctors are now prescribing it as well.

TREATING INSULIN RESISTANCE

Weight loss is one of the simplest, yet most effective, ways to manage insulin abnormalities, menstrual irregularities, and other PCOS symptoms. For weight-loss strategies, see Chapter 11.

Insulin-lowering drugs are another option. This class of drugs includes the diabetes drug metformin (Glucophage). Metformin has been receiving a lot of media attention and has been brilliantly effective for some women with PCOS.

In preliminary studies,[7] metformin helped restore normal menstrual cycles in approximately 50 per cent of women with PCOS. Blood androgen (male hormone) levels sometimes also decrease, but there may not be much improvement in excess hair growth or acne. And metformin doesn't provide contraception. In fact, it might stimulate ovulation – great if you do want to conceive, not so great if you don't!

Metformin may also help with weight loss, though it's not a weight-loss drug. Some studies[8] have shown that women with PCOS on a low-calorie diet lose more weight when metformin is added. But to keep the weight off you need to stick to a healthy eating and exercise plan; otherwise it creeps back on.

There's also been speculation that metformin might reduce the risk of early pregnancy loss and the development of gestational diabetes mellitus (diabetes during pregnancy) in women with PCOS. But experts don't yet recommend its use in these situations until larger studies have been undertaken.

Metformin is available in three forms:

1. Generic Metformin Hcl
2. Glucophage (brand name)
3. Glucophage XR (brand name).

Glucophage is available in 500-mg, 850-mg or 1,000-mg tablets. The usual dose is 850–1,000mg twice daily. Your doctor will probably help you to build up to the appropriate dose gradually.

Side-effects can include diarrhoea and more frequent bowel movements – and some women feel this is why they've lost weight while they've been using it, and the reason why it's all gone back on again once they've got used to the medication. But every case is individual and you'd work with your doctor to find the best dose for you.

The long-term safety and effectiveness of metformin and other experimental drugs for PCOS is still unknown.

'My doctor agreed to start me on 500mg of Metformin twice daily, and we built up to 850mg, then 1,000mg. At this level I noticed a metallic taste in my mouth … I went back to the 850mg dose. I have started to lose weight and have had two periods in the last 3½ months,

Janey, 32

FERTILITY TREATMENT

If you're finding it hard to get pregnant your doctor will usually ask both you and your partner to have a thorough check-up. These exams may include tests of the fallopian tubes in the woman and a semen analysis in the man. If tests determine that the problem is lack of ovulation due to PCOS, three options are available. It's important to know that all of these options work best for women who aren't obese, and that even a modest amount of weight loss can make these treatments more effective.

CLOMIPHENE CITRATE

The first line of treatment is typically the fertility drug clomiphene citrate, which stimulates the ovaries to release one or more eggs. Clomiphene triggers ovulation in about 80 per cent of women with PCOS, and about 50 per cent of these women will actually become pregnant. In women taking clomiphene, ovulation can be confirmed by blood and urine tests or by measurement of body temperature. If the original dose of clomiphene does not trigger ovulation, the doctor may prescribe a higher dose.

Several studies[9] have shown that the insulin-sensitizing drug, metformin, increases the effectiveness of clomiphene in producing ovulation. And another study[10] suggested metformin may reduce the risk of miscarriage. So your specialist may prescribe it alongside clomiphene.

Although many women use metformin in their pursuit of a successful pregnancy, and early studies[11] look promising, it's important to point out that its safety for use during pregnancy has not been firmly established.

Metformin does contribute to increased homocysteine levels, and increased homocysteine levels can increase the risk of miscarriage.

GONADOTROPIN THERAPY

A more aggressive medical treatment for PCOS-related infertility is with drugs called gonadotropins (LH and FSH). FSH is used without LH for women with PCOS, and is given as a daily injection for 7 to 10 days. These drugs trigger ovulation in almost all women with PCOS and lead to pregnancy in approximately 60 per cent. But these drugs are expensive; they can also overstimulate the ovaries and produce pregnancy with multiple foetuses because lots of eggs are ready to be fertilised at the same time.

OVARIAN SURGERY

Surgery is only used as a last measure for the treatment of infertility in women with PCOS, but can be effective in some women who do not respond to medical treatment.

Today, surgery is usually performed through a laparoscope (a thin, lighted tube). Instruments are inserted through the laparoscope and are used to damage the ovary mechanically or thermally (with heat or cold). This damage decreases androgen levels in the ovary and alters other hormonc levels in the body, triggering the maturation and release of eggs.

Women with PCOS have an 80 to 87 per cent chance of becoming pregnant after laparoscopic surgery, and it usually reinstates normal menstrual cycles for at least several months afterwards. But it's not without risks – it's typically less effective in overweight women, and can lead to the formation of adhesions, wasting of the ovary, injury to surrounding tissues, and infection. Although the long-term effects of ovarian surgery are still being evaluated, studies suggest that the procedure may also lead to early menopause.

FUTURE RESEARCH

Research on PCOS and clinical trials addressing the best treatments are taking place in many countries around the world.

At the time of writing there's currently a lot of research in the area of genetics as regards PCOS and the best way to treat it. Micro-rays are miniature chips that permit the screening of thousands and thousands of genes, and this type of research is simplifying the search for genes that have an impact on ovarian function, insulin resistance and PCOS.

With the increasing interest in hormonal therapies for prostate cancer it's likely that novel treatments for the PCOS symptoms of hirsutism and acne will one day be found, such as a pure anti-androgen that has an effect only on the skin and doesn't upset the menstrual cycle.

Preliminary research is also looking at the widely available anti-cholesterol drug simvastatin as a treatment for PCOS. Researchers at Yale University School of Medicine studied 48 women with PCOS. Levels of testosterone fell by an average of 18 per cent and cholesterol by 12 per cent in the women taking simvastatin. It also reduced hirsutism by 4 per cent and helped some women get rid of acne. Those who took part in the trial took twice the normal 10-mg dose usually recommended for cholesterol-lowering effect. More research needs to be done.

Several large-scale studies are underway to determine metformin's safety and effectiveness for use in the long term and during pregnancy. Other studies are attempting, among other things, to determine why the ovaries are sensitive to insulin, what the most effective diet is for women with PCOS, and the impact of weight loss, diet and lifestyle on symptoms.

One other insulin-sensitizing medication, inositol,[12] is showing particular promise. It will be a while before conclusions can be drawn, but at present one thing is certain: the now accepted link between PCOS and insulin resistance and diabetes has ensured that PCOS will never again be neglected by the medical community. The search for new treatment options will continue.

WHERE TO GO FROM HERE

Now you've seen what's on offer from the medical community you need to decide how best to work with your doctor, weigh up the pros and cons and find a treatment approach that's best for you. Whether or not you decide to go down the medical route, it's absolutely vital that you give yourself and your medication, if you're taking it, a helping hand by making some positive lifestyle changes. Study after study[13] has confirmed that a good diet, exercise programme and lifestyle modification are the *essential* foundation in managing PCOS. In some cases these may even be all you need to manage your symptoms, but if you're on medication your goal should always be to use it in conjunction with diet and exercise, as the healthier you are the more effective your medication is likely to be.

This is why Part 2 is packed with practical diet and lifestyle advice that can help you beat your symptoms, reduce the long-term health risks associated with PCOS and boost your chances of health and vitality, now and in the years to come.

PART TWO
TOTAL TLC FOR YOUR BODY: ACTION PLAN FOR YOUR HEALTH NOW AND IN THE FUTURE

CHAPTER 6
YOUR PCOS NUTRITION GUIDE

To truly get to grips with PCOS, you have to eat the foods that are right for you. Dozens of medical studies[1] have shown that eating the right kinds of foods can help manage symptoms and reduce the risk of infertility, diabetes, heart disease and other complications of PCOS.

WHY FOOD IS SO IMPORTANT FOR PCOS

1. Food influences your hormones. Everything you put in your mouth triggers some kind of hormonal response in your body.
2. A healthy diet plays a vital role in weight management. Study after study[2] has shown that how much you weigh is one of the most significant factors in determining how severe your symptoms are.

3. You have to eat – so food is a natural medicine you can access for yourself. And taking control of your diet can get rid of feelings of powerlessness in the face of PCOS.

4. The nutrients in your food actually become the cells of your body – we are what we eat. Nutritional deficiencies – when you don't get enough of all the essential nutrients and vitamins and minerals you need for good health – are caused by stress and a poor diet. They can upset your body's hormonal balance, your mood and your long-term health.

5. Eating right could alter your genetics – and protect your kids from PCOS. Research is still preliminary, but in the November 2005 issue of *New Scientist*[3] journal, experts drew on a number of studies on animals to suggest that a person's diet could in theory have an impact on their genetic make-up. This means that genetic effects which predispose people to have physical or mental illness could be switched 'on' or 'off', according to the food you eat, and could possibly reverse the effects of diseases such as schizophrenia or cancer.

6. A good diet makes medication more effective. For example, Gerard Conway, consultant gynaecologist at Middlesex Hospital, says 'Metformin is not a magic bullet and will only work if a foundation of healthy eating and exercise is already in place.'

THE 10-STEP PCOS DIET ACTION PLAN

A balanced, nutritious, whole food, low-glycaemic diet can have the most positive effect on women with PCOS,[4] easing their symptoms and reducing the long-term health risks, so here's the simplest way to get it.

Be sure to give yourself time to adjust to the PCOS diet. If you're used to eating in a certain way, it will take time to re-educate your taste buds. A whole new diet introduced all at once could also shock your system and trigger fatigue, headaches and stomach upsets. It's much better to make gradual changes and to train your palate and your digestion slowly. It takes most people about three to four months to adjust to a new eating plan, and that's what we recommend.

Each of the ten changes will make a huge difference and encourage you to make even more. From our own personal experience and from talking to other women with PCOS, the order in which we have listed our plan makes for the easiest way to start incorporating the stages into your life. Try each change and stick with it for a couple of days or weeks, or however long you need to feel comfortable with it before moving on to the next one.

Think of the changes not as rules but as guidelines for a lifetime of healthy eating that you can use to ensure your body gets all the nutrients it needs to beat your symptoms and boost the quality of your health and your life. The menu planners and meal ideas on pages 96–100 show that making changes doesn't have to be complicated!

1) EAT MORE OFTEN

The PCOS diet is about eating more, not less, as long as those foods are healthy and nutritious. It's also about eating more often. Try not to go more than three or four hours without eating. Most of us find ourselves skipping breakfast or grabbing a coffee, followed by a light lunch and then an evening meal which can be as late as 9 or 10 p.m. Starving and stacking your calories like this just isn't a good idea if you have PCOS.

WHY?

When you fast for long periods your body thinks starvation is on the horizon and responds by doing the best it can to hold on to every calorie by reducing your metabolic rate and preparing to store fat.

Long gaps between meals also create low blood sugar levels, which make you crave sugary foods and snacks – the very foods that cause a surge of insulin and add to the likelihood of insulin resistance.

HOW?

Have breakfast, a mid-morning snack, lunch, an afternoon snack and then a light supper.

Breakfast is your most important meal because it kick-starts your metabolism, gives you an energy boost and gets you going for the day. If you don't feel like eating when you get up, try waking up 15 minutes earlier or laying the breakfast table the evening before to motivate you.

Your snacks should be a low-GI carbohydrate mixed with a little protein. Points 3 and 5 below will explain why this is important, but for now the healthy PCOS snack suggestions opposite will help get you thinking along the right lines.

Make sure you have a good lunch and only a light supper so you eat most of your calories early in the day when you have a chance to use them up by being active. If you eat a big evening meal, then go to bed, you'll just store away the calories, confuse your metabolic rate and put on weight.

⇨ HEALTHY SNACK IDEAS

- Crisp vegetable sticks with peanut dipping sauce.
- Celery sticks filled with cottage cheese and topped with sultanas or chopped nuts.
- Raw vegetables, such as celery, carrots, cauliflower, broccoli, green pepper, green beans, cucumbers, mushrooms or zucchini with a low-fat hummus dip.
- A handful of nuts and/or seeds with fresh fruit in season, cut in slices or halves, such as apples, oranges, bananas, peaches, grapefruit, grapes, melons, pears, plums or strawberries.
- A mixture of low-fat hard cheese cubes with nuts and dried fruits.
- Thin slices of carrot and celery rolled up and filled with low-fat grated cheese and a slice of cold meat.
- Next time you're making meatloaf, double the quantity and make a batch of meatballs. These are great little snacks. Add a slice of pineapple with a toothpick to each meatball. You could even add tomato dipping sauce.
- Make a batch of crust-less quiche and cook it in a muffin tray for healthy bites. This tastes delicious with wholegrain mustard.
- Try wholewheat crackers spread with mashed banana and cinnamon, or mashed avocado, sliced tomato and beansprouts.
- Chopped hard-boiled egg with low-fat mayo, herbs (e.g. basil) and spices (e.g. paprika) on a crispbread.
- Wrap a cheese finger, celery stick and carrot stick in a lettuce leaf.
- Plain yoghurt topped with nuts and seeds (0% fat Greek yoghurt feels like a treat, and also tastes great with chopped fruit).
- Fresh chicken breast wrapped in several sheets of thin pastry. Brush pastry with beaten egg to glaze. Cut into desired lengths and bake in a moderately hot oven for 15–20 minutes. Use tomato or your favourite dipping sauce.

- Spread a round of pitta bread with tomato paste and herbs. Top with tomato, ham, mortadella, onion, sliced mushrooms or pineapple. Sprinkle with grated low-fat hard cheese and grill to make a tasty mini pizza.
- Place bite-sized pieces of fruit in season on kebab skewers and sprinkle with seeds or toasted pine nuts.

2) GO FOR WHOLE FOODS

Whole food means unrefined foods in their most natural form – vegetables, fruits, oats, wholemeal bread, wholewheat pasta and brown rice – which are naturally full of vitamins and minerals. Whole foods do not contain any additives such as artificial flavourings, colourings or preservatives.

WHY?

Whole foods are bursting with goodness because they've had none of their nutrients or fibre taken away and no chemicals have been added. Your body loves whole foods because it can absorb all that goodness easily without having to work through all the junk at the same time.

As well as being packed with nutrients your body needs for good health, whole foods contain plenty of fibre, or roughage, which has a stimulating effect on the digestive system. A diet rich in fibre is particularly therapeutic for women with PCOS because fibre is thought to prevent excess oestrogen from being reabsorbed into the blood.[5]

A high-fibre diet can also reduce the risk of insulin resistance by slowing down the conversion of carbohydrates into blood sugar.[6]

HOW?

Fresh vegetables, fresh fruits, wholegrain cereals and breads, legumes (peas and beans), fresh fish, nuts and seeds are all whole foods, so eat more of them. Choose brown pasta, wholegrain bread, wholegrain cereals, and eat lots of fresh fruit and veg. Try always to have fresh soups, smoothies and juices (not made from concentrates), and eat a side salad with every meal. Snack on fruit as well, and you're well on the way to eating more wholefoods.

Avoid refined flours and bran as they have little nutritional value and act too fast, preventing you from absorbing nutrients. Healthy flours include wholemeal, quinoa, maize, rye, oat, barley, wheat germ and brown rice. Buckwheat and millet aren't strictly speaking grains, but they make good alternatives.

Legumes, such as peas and beans (great in soups, stews, casseroles and dips like hummus), are another good source of fibre. Drink plenty of water to help whole foods pass through your system efficiently. And if you aren't used to a whole-food high-fibre diet, you need to introduce it slowly to give your digestive system and your bowels time to adjust.

▷ SAMPLE WHOLE FOOD MENU

- *Breakfast:* Oat porridge with chopped fruit.
- *Mid-morning Smoothie:* 10 fl oz (285 ml) goat's milk, a banana and 3 oz (100 g) raspberries or strawberries.
- *Lunch:* Hummus or lean chicken with salad, tomato and onion on wholegrain bread plus an apple and a few walnuts.
- *Mid-afternoon:* Low-fat yoghurt with a handful of nuts and seeds.
- *Dinner:* Wholegrain rice with lean fish, vegetables and a green bean salad, plus a fruit salad for dessert.

3) MONITOR YOUR SUGAR INTAKE

Once you've got used to eating regularly and having more whole foods, you're more than ready for the next phase: monitoring your sugar intake.

WHY?

Eating more sugar than your body needs has been linked to many health problems, from diabetes to heart disease, obesity to cancer and, of course, PCOS. Sugar has no nutrients but lots of calories, and it goes straight to your bloodstream where it raises blood sugar levels, stimulates the release of insulin, triggers PCOS symptoms, contributes to weight gain and depresses the immune system so you're more likely to get constant colds.

Sugar does have one thing going for it – it gives you energy. But your body gets plenty of sugar from whole foods such as fruits and unrefined carbohydrates; you don't need to get it from the sugar bowl or from cakes, sweets or pastries.

We're not suggesting you cut out sweets altogether, but you do need to monitor your sugar intake and cut down. Don't forget that once the sugar has been digested it turns into FAT, something most women with PCOS don't want or need.

HOW?

Most of the sugar we eat is hidden in our foods – not just in cakes and sweets but in juice drinks, sodas and refined, processed, pre-packaged foods from cheese slices and crisps to breakfast cereals, pre-packed pasta sauces and pickles.

It's easy to cut down on sugar by cutting down on sweets, biscuits, cakes, pies, doughnuts and other processed refined foods with added sugar.

Start reading labels on your favourite foods. You may be surprised at how much sugar you discover there, in one of its many disguises: sucrose, raw sugar, brown sugar, turbinado sugar, sucrose, dextrose, honey, lactose, invert sugar, confectioner's sugar, corn syrup, fructose, glucose, sorbitol, mannitol, malitol, treacle, molasses and so on. The higher up the sugar is listed, the more there is in the product.

Are any of these sugars better than the others? No. Forget the fancy names. The bottom line is 'sugar is sugar' – and in any form it's high in calories and low in nutrients. Honey offers no special health benefits, either (unless you smooth it on to sunburned or dry skin as a natural face mask!).

Eat fresh fruit or choose low-fat low-sugar muffins or dried fruit. Go for oat or wholegrain breakfast cereals that contain no more than 5 g of sugar per serving. Make batches of your own pasta sauce and freeze them. And look at what you're drinking – sodas and fruit drinks are often very high in sugar. Most popular brands contain only about 10 per cent juice, so try watering these down with spring water or choose freshly pressed juice and add water.

After a while you may find that your body starts to lose its taste for sugar and you don't even miss it. (If you've ever given up having sugar in your tea you'll know what we mean here.) It's the same with cutting down on sugar in all your food – the more you cut down, the less you hanker for it.

Sugar substitutes and sweeteners aren't much better if you've got PCOS – they've been linked to stomach upsets, hormonal problems, headaches and even weight gain and cancer.[7] If you really need some sweetness, a tiny pinch of sugar is OK, but far better to add natural sweeteners like fruit juice or fresh fruit. The herbal alternative Stevia, available from most health food stores, is sweet tasting, calorie free and worth checking out.

4) MAKE THE GLYCAEMIC FACTOR WORK FOR YOU

If you're eating more delicious whole foods and are cutting down on sugar, you're definitely ready to be introduced to the glycaemic factor.

WHY?

The glycaemic index was originally designed for people with diabetes to help them keep their blood sugar levels under control. Since improvement in PCOS symptoms is associated with blood sugar imbalance, the glycaemic index (GI) can be a very useful tool for us.

The GI ranks food by the influence they have on your blood sugar levels a few hours after you eat them. Glucose is used as the reference food and its index value is set at 100. All other foods are then compared to glucose and ranked accordingly.

Foods that have a GI of 70 or more are typically called 'high glycaemic index foods' as they trigger a rapid rise in blood sugar. Foods with a GI of 55 to 69 are called 'medium glycaemic index foods' as they trigger a moderate increase. Foods with a GI below 55 are called 'low glycaemic foods' because they have only a moderate to low impact on blood sugar.

There are plenty of books and websites which list the glycaemic value of various foods (see Resources) but the following should help you stick to the basic principles.

Foods that are white tend to have a high glycaemic index. This includes processed foods made with white flour and white sugar – but even white potatoes have a high GI. If you're sticking to change Number 3 (moderating your sugar intake) you should be doing this already.

Concentrate on eating foods that are high in fibre (you'll be doing this already if you're choosing whole foods). In general, high-fibre foods take longer to digest and therefore produce a slower rise in blood glucose levels. Fibre also keeps you feeling fuller for longer, which helps prevent overeating. Most vegetables, whole grains, legumes, nuts, seeds, and even fruits such as apples and pears are rich in fibre when you eat them whole (not as juice).

USING THE GI FOR PCOS

The GI alone is not the best way to determine how PCOS-friendly a food is. For example, ice cream and sponge cake are listed as low GI because they're high in fat, and fat slows down the speed at which your body releases sugar – but these foods are also low in nutrients and high in calories. You'll also find that some highly nutritious foods, rich in vitamins and minerals, such as carrots and parsnips are high on the GI because they convert to sugar quickly. But given the choice between carrot sticks or ice cream for a snack, it's not rocket science to work out which is healthier!

THINK ABOUT YOUR WHOLE MEAL

Your glycaemic response to a food also depends on the other foods you eat with it. You can eat healthy high-GI foods such as carrots or parsnips in a meal that also contains fibre, protein and essential fats which slow down the speed at which your body releases sugar from your meal.

For example, have a high-GI baked potato with low-fat cheese (protein) and a green salad (fibre), or higher-GI carrot soup sprinkled with seeds (essential fats) and whole grain pitta (fibre) stuffed with lean chicken (protein). That way you'll get all the nutrients from healthy high-GI foods while minimizing the effect on your blood sugar.

THINK ABOUT GLYCAEMIC LOAD

Another great thing to think about is portion size – because the total amount of insulin your body produces depends not just on a food's GI but also on its carbohydrate density – also known as the glycaemic load.

The GI only reflects how quickly a food raises blood sugar levels – it doesn't take into account how much of that food makes up an average portion. And the amount of carbs in an average portion is what actually goes into your body on a day-to-day basis – so this is what the *GL* measures: *the glycaemic effect of an average portion of a food.* The GL of a food is obtained by dividing the GI value by 100, then multiplying by the amount of total carbohydrate per typical serving of the food.

A low-GL food is considered 10 or less, medium 11–19 and high would be 20 or more.

The great thing about this is that a food that can come up high on the GI table might actually come out low on the GL, because you wouldn't eat enough of it in an average portion to send your blood sugar soaring.

For example, carrots have a glycaemic index value of 92 which is high. But, in a typical serving size of one-half cup, there's only 4.2 grams of carbohydrate. So, the calculated GL is only 3.9, which is very low, showing that this food is unlikely to cause a disturbance in blood sugar or insulin response. By contrast, a plain bagel provides 65 grams of carbohydrate and has a GI of 73. Its glycaemic load is therefore a massive 47.

The following chart will help you identify both the GI and GL of commonly eaten foods.

⟳ GLYCAEMIC INDEXES AND LOADS FOR COMMON FOODS

The table below shows values of the Glycaemic Index (GI) and Glycaemic Load (GL) for a few common foods. GIs of 55 or below are considered low, and 70 or above are considered high. GLs of 10 or below are considered low, and 20 or above are considered high.

Food	GI	Serving Size	Net Carbs	GL
Peanuts	14	4 oz (113g)	15	2
Bean sprouts	25	1 cup (104g)	4	1
Grapefruit	25	½ large (166g)	11	3
Pizza	30	2 slices (260g)	42	13
Low-fat yoghurt	33	1 cup (245g)	47	16
Apples	38	1 medium (138g)	16	6
Spaghetti	42	1 cup (140g)	38	16
Carrots	47	1 large (72g)	5	2
Oranges	48	1 medium (131g)	12	6
Bananas	52	1 large (136g)	27	14
Potato chips	54	4 oz (114g)	55	30

Food	GI	Serving Size	Net Carbs	GL
Snickers Bar	55	1 bar (113g)	64	35
Brown rice	55	1 cup (195g)	42	23
Honey	55	1 tbsp (21g)	17	9
Oatmeal	58	1 cup (234g)	21	12
Ice cream	61	1 cup (72g)	16	10
Macaroni and cheese	64	1 serving (166g)	47	30
Raisins	64	1 small box (43g)	32	20
White rice	64	1 cup (186g)	52	33
Sugar (sucrose)	68	1 tbsp (12g)	12	8
White bread	70	1 slice (30g)	14	10
Watermelon	72	1 cup (154g)	11	8
Popcorn	72	2 cups (16g)	10	7
Baked potato	85	1 medium (173g)	33	28
Glucose	100	(50g)	50	50

LEARNING MORE

Additional information and values for Glycaemic Index and Glycaemic Load can be found at www.glycaemicindex.com and http://www.mendosa.com/gilists.htm

Also bear in mind that the cooking process will alter the glycaemic value of a meal. Generally, the longer food is cooked (or processed), the higher the glycaemic value. It's also worth knowing that adding protein, fibre, healthy fat or acid (such as vinegar or lemon juice) to food will generally lower glycaemic values.

LOW GI AND PCOS – IN A NUTSHELL

What all this really tells you is that whole foods are your best food choice, and if you think a food has a high GI watch your portion size and eat some protein and fibre with it.

Rather than selecting foods solely based on their GI or GL, we'd far rather you concentrated on eating a balanced diet and enjoyed your food. Use your common sense and evaluate foods for their overall health value. If you do choose to plan your diet using the GI or GL as a guide, look at food values for an entire day rather than excluding a food because it has a high value, and aim to keep your GL to 80 per day. When you eat foods with a high GI, the smaller the serving size, the smaller the rise in your blood sugar and insulin response. Foods with a high GI but low GL can be included as part of a healthy diet. Foods with a low GI will always have a low GL.

Use the GI and GL by all means if you want to, but don't get carried away with calculations for every meal you eat. If you can't get your head around the GI and GL, it won't spell disaster for your PCOS diet. Whether you work with the GI or not, the best way to make PCOS-friendly food choices is to follow the first three recommendations of our PCOS diet and replace processed and refined foods (sweets, cakes, white bread and sugar) with whole foods such as fresh fruits, vegetables, whole grains, legumes, nuts and seeds.

▷ SAMPLE GI-/GL-FRIENDLY MENU
- *Breakfast:* Oat porridge
- *Mid-morning snack:* Smoothie – 10oz goat's milk, 1 banana, 3oz berries
- *Lunch:* Hummus or lean chicken with salad, tomato and onion on wholegrain bread; an apple; a few walnuts

- *Mid-afternoon snack:* Low fat yoghurt; nuts and seeds
- *Dinner:* Wholegrain rice with lean fish, vegetables, green bean salad; fruit salad

5) DRINK MORE WATER

Cutting down on sugar and working out the glycaemic factor of your diet are probably the hardest and most challenging changes we'll be asking you to make. It really does get easier from now on. Change Number 5, for example, is simple: drink more water.

WHY?

Not only is your body two-thirds water, but water intake and distribution are essential for hormonal balance. Water also helps your body metabolize stored fat by maximizing muscle function, so is also crucial for weight management. Water regulates body temperature and provides the means for nutrients to travel to all your organs, as well as transporting oxygen to our cells, removing waste and protecting our joints and organs.

Water may also help reduce the increased risk of heart disease and high blood pressure associated with PCOS. Research[8] suggests that people who drink five or more 8-ounce (225-ml) glasses of water a day have fewer heart attacks than those who drink two or fewer glasses. This is because dehydration seems to increase the tendency for blood to clot, and blood-clotting is a risk factor for heart disease.

SIGNS OF DEHYDRATION

We lose water through urination, respiration and by sweating. Diuretics such as caffeine and alcohol result in the need to drink more water because they trick our bodies into thinking we have more water than we need.

Symptoms of mild dehydration include chronic pains in joints and muscles, lower back pain, headaches and constipation. A strong odour to your urine, along with a yellow or amber colour, indicates that you're not getting enough water. Thirst is an obvious sign of dehydration, though in fact you need water long before you feel thirsty.

HOW MUCH?

On average you should try to drink eight 8-ounce (225-ml) glasses of water a day. A good rule of thumb is to take your body weight in pounds and divide that number in half. That gives you the number of ounces of water per day that you need to drink. If you exercise you should drink another 8-ounce glass of water for every 20 minutes you are active. If you drink coffee or alcohol, you should drink at least an equal amount of water. When you're travelling on an airplane, it's good to drink 8 ounces of water for every hour you're on board the plane. If you live in an arid climate or are always near central heating, you should add another two glasses per day.

As you can see, your daily need for water can add up to quite a lot.

The best source of water is plain, pure drinking water. Fizzy drinks have a lot of sugar in them and aren't a good source, so if you drink them, they won't count towards your daily amount. Herbal teas that aren't diuretic are fine (steer clear of dandelion, parsley, nettle and fennel). Sports drinks contain electrolytes and may be beneficial, just look out for added sugar and calories that you don't need.

If you aren't sure you're drinking enough, keep a record for a few days. Any non-caffeinated, non-fizzy drinks can be counted as fluid. If you aren't drinking enough, here are some ideas for including more fluids:

- Carry a water bottle. It may be difficult to drink enough water on a busy day. Be sure you have water handy at all times by keeping a bottle with you when you're working, travelling or exercising.
- Add some lemon. If you get bored with plain water, add a bit of lemon or lime for a touch of flavour. There are some brands of flavoured water available, but some of them have sugar or artificial sweeteners which you don't need.
- Experiment with herbal teas, watered-down fruit juices or diluted fresh-pressed juice – but watch out for juice drinks that are loaded with sugar.
- Drink fluids at room temperature. You wouldn't water your plants with freezing cold water or put icy water into your pet's water bowl, would you? In Traditional Chinese Medicine, cold drinks disrupt the proper flow of energy in the body and 'shock' the body. Stick to warm or room-temperature fluids.

As a rule of thumb, filtered water is best. Tap water can be contaminated with heavy metals, micro-organisms, chlorine, fluoride and other impurities. Still, if bottled water proves too expensive, tap water will do just fine, especially if you use a water filter.

If you're eating plenty of fruits and vegetables this will count towards your fluid intake, as they are 90 per cent water.

6) PASS ON THE SALT

The next stage on the PCOS diet is to cut down on salt. Instead of adding salt to your food, add herbs, spices or lemon juice for flavour.

WHY?

A diet high in salt can increase your already higher risk of high blood pressure and cause fluid retention.

HOW?

First of all, get out of the habit of adding salt to your food and your cooking and experiment with herbs, spices, lemon juice, mustard powder, lime juice, vinegar, red or wine white, onions, garlic, ginger, chillies, etc.

If you've always added salt to your food this may be tough, but once you get used to cutting back you'll discover all those wonderful and more subtle flavours that were drowned out by the overpowering taste of salt. If you really can't get used to not having salt with some foods, try a salt substitute such as LoSalt which contains potassium instead of sodium.

You also need to be aware that salt is a hidden ingredient in many foods, in particular processed and pre-packed foods, so once again you need to read labels to check for salt (sodium) content. To find out how much salt is in a food, multiply the sodium content on the label by 2.5. You should aim for fewer than 5 g of salt a day.

You also need to avoid foods such as cured and smoked meats, smoked and pickled fish, tinned meats, salted nuts, salted butter, biscuits, beans and vegetables in brine. Go instead for low-salt alternatives such as fresh fish, fresh lean meat, unsalted butter and nuts, dried fruit, beans and vegetables frozen with no added salt, olives in oil and low-salt versions of sauces.

1. Read food labels to choose foods lower in sodium.
2. Eat fewer canned and processed foods that are high in sodium (e.g., bologna, crisp pork rinds, sausage, pepperoni, salami, hot dogs, tinned and instant soups, cheese, and chips).
3. Eat fresh fruits and vegetables instead of salty snacks.
4. Eat fewer salted crackers and nuts. Try unsalted nuts and unsalted or low-sodium crackers.
5. Eat fewer olives and pickles.
6. Use half the amount of salt you normally use when cooking, if any.
7. Better still, cook and season food with herbs and spices instead of salt.
8. Use less bouillon, adobo, capers and soy sauce. If you use these condiments, do not add salt to your food. Use garlic powder and onion powder instead of garlic salt or onion salt.
9. Take the salt cellar off the table.
10. If you're eating out, ask that salt not be added to your portion.

7) EAT THE RIGHT FATS

Next it's time to swap bad fats for good fats in your PCOS diet action plan.

WHY?

There are bad fats that can increase your risk of health complications due to PCOS, and good fats that can protect you from the symptoms of PCOS.

Saturated fats are the 'bad' fats found in dairy products and red meat. These animal fats are bad for us because they contain unhealthy prostaglandins (which can trigger blood-clotting) and hormones and antibiotics that can upset your digestive, immune and hormonal systems. If that weren't enough, saturated fats can cause weight gain, interfere with the absorption of other nutrients and stimulate oestrogen production.

You also need to avoid hydrogenated fats and oils in the form of fried, oxidized or trans fats found in margarines, vegetable shortenings and many processed foods and fast food snacks as well as cakes, sweets and biscuits. These vegetable oils contain transfatty acids that can increase your risk of diabetes and heart disease.[9]

But you shouldn't avoid fat altogether — because the right fats can protect your health.

Unsaturated fats[10] (polyunsaturated and monounsaturated) have a protective effect on the heart and are found in olive oil and foods such as avocado, but the most beneficial fats for women with PCOS are the Omega 3 essential fats and, to a lesser extent, the Omega 6 fats. You can find both these fats in oily fish, nuts and seeds. Every single cell in your body needs these essential fats (EFAs) to maintain the cell wall so it's flexible enough to take in nutrients and push out toxins. They are also crucial for hormone balance, weight-management and fertility.

EFAs help protect your heart by helping your body make the healthy kind of prostaglandins that can help reduce the risk of blood-clotting. (Some experts also believe that, as EFAs are needed in your cell membranes, they don't travel to fat cells in your bum and thighs because your body uses them.) A diet low in EFAs can make PCOS symptoms worse and increase the risk of insulin resistance, weight gain and heart disease.[11] This is because EFAs delay the passage of carbohydrates in your system and keep blood sugar levels stable and insulin levels down. EFAs are without doubt one of the best blood sugar-stabilizers, and as you're well aware a stable blood sugar means a reduction in symptoms and less likelihood of obesity, diabetes, heart disease and even depression.

A low-fat diet is wrong for women with PCOS – we need fat. But, as with carbohydrates, we need to make sure we're eating the right kind.

HOW?

To limit your intake of saturated fats, choose low-fat dairy products, spreads, white meat and fish and lean cuts of red meat.

Transfatty acids are harder to avoid than saturated fats because they're hidden in margarines, processed foods and snack foods such as biscuits, cakes and crisps. If you're upping your intake of whole foods and fibre and cutting down on sugar and refined carbohydrates, you may already have cut down on the transfats. Instead of margarine it might be better to go for a small amount of spreadable butter.

Increase your intake of Omega 6 and Omega 3. You're less likely to be deficient in Omega 6 because it's more common in Western diets and found in foods such as leafy green vegetables and soy, olive, sunflower and sesame oils. Omega 3s are less common and found in the oils of cold-water fish (such as mackerel, salmon, herring and sardines) as well as in hemp seeds, flaxseeds, soy oil, nuts and seeds.

Aim to eat oily fish at least twice a week, but not more than four times a week. If you don't eat fish you can eat sea vegetables (sea weeds) and up your intake of hemp seeds and flaxseeds. Flaxseeds and hemp seeds are a great source of Omega 3. You might like to try a daily dose of 3 teaspoons of cold-pressed flaxseed oil or 3 tablespoons of ground flaxseed. You can also use hemp and flaxseeds in salad dressings and smoothies or sprinkled on cereals.

Use only cold-pressed vegetable oils. Of the readily available vegetable oils, only three contain both Omega 3 and Omega 6: flaxseed, hempseed and soy oil, so aim to use these. Other oils such as olive and sunflower do contain Omega 6, but not enough Omega 3.

Nuts such as walnuts, almonds, pecans, brazils and cashews, and seeds such as pumpkin, sunflower, hemp and sesame are good sources of EFAs, so try to eat a handful every day, perhaps as a snack between meals or sprinkled on your salads, soups or cereals. You can also use them in baking.

Finally, avoiding processed and refined foods is a great way to ensure you get more EFAs in your diet, as highly processed foods block the absorption of EFAs.

▷ SAMPLE 'GOOD FAT' MENU

- *Breakfast:* Fruit salad or smoothie with ground flaxseed
- *Mid-morning snack:* Banana and handful of sunflower, hemp, pumpkin and sesame seeds
- *Lunch:* Salmon served with new potatoes and a large serving of green vegetables
- *Mid-afternoon snack:* Glass of skimmed milk; handful nuts
- *Dinner:* Pasta in tomato sauce served with salad; low-fat, low-sugar yoghurt with sprinkling of cinnamon and walnut

8) GIVE YOURSELF A DAILY PROTEIN CHECK

You should aim to eat a diet that's around 50 per cent carbohydrate (whole foods and low GI, of course), 20 to 25 per cent healthy fats, and 20 to 25 per cent good-quality protein. We've covered carbohydrates and fat already; now the spotlight turns on proteins.

WHY?

A daily protein check is important because, as we've seen, protein plays an important role in maintaining blood sugar balance. If you eat it with a sugary or high-GI food it will slow down the conversion of sugar. Protein also supplies the amino acids our bodies need to build and repair cells and manufacture hormones and brain chemicals. And it helps to break down stored fat for use as fuel, which helps keep insulin levels down. Our bodies can't store protein as they can carbohydrate and fat, so you need a constant supply.

HOW?

Too much protein isn't wise if you have PCOS because it leaves less room for all the other nutrient-rich carbohydrates and fats that we need to balance our blood sugar and boost our energy. So we're not recommending a high-protein diet here – especially as it can lead to an increased risk of diabetes and heart disease and perhaps trigger insulin resistance. That's why we recommend that you eat some good-quality protein with every meal while making sure you also eat the right kind of nutritious and healthy carbs and fats as part of a varied and balanced diet. Include a range of low-fat protein in your diet and make sure that you have a serving with every meal – try low-fat cheese, low-fat milk, low-fat yoghurt, lean meat, poultry, seafood, fish, nuts and seeds.

Other great sources of protein include soybeans, peas, kidney beans, wheat germ, lima beans, black-eyed peas, chickpeas, lentils, black beans, soy products, tofu products, quinoa (a seed that you cook like couscous or rice), spirulina (a green powdered algae you get from health stores to sprinkle in shakes or smoothies, or which you can get in capsule form) and quorn (a meat substitute made from mushroom protein).

Eggs are also a good idea – especially organic, free-range ones. You should try to eat at least two or three eggs a week for their protein and lecithin – a kind of biological 'detergent' that can help break down fats, detox your blood and transport of nutrients through the cell walls. (Eggs should be soft boiled or poached, since a hard yolk binds the lecithin and limits its action.)

Skimmed milk also has the benefit of protecting against high blood pressure.[12]

PROTEINS FOR VEGETARIANS AND VEGANS

People choose a vegetarian diet for religious, ethical, health or environmental reasons. A vegetarian diet generally contains less total fat, saturated fat and cholesterol, and includes more dietary fibre. And vegetarians tend to have lower rates of some cancers, cardiovascular disease, high blood pressure and Type 2 diabetes.

Adopting a healthy vegetarian diet means substituting meat with a vegetarian protein source, and eat a varied diet including around 30 g of nuts and seeds a day and around 3 or 4 soft boiled eggs a week. The advice below should help you make sure you meet your daily nutritional needs.

Vegetarian Sources of Protein

Eggs

Cheese

Milk

Yoghurt

Vegan Sources of Protein

Leafy green vegetables, including spinach

Legumes – beans, lentils, peas, peanuts

Nuts – almonds, walnuts, cashews, etc.

Seaweed – kelp, spirulina, etc.

Seeds – sesame, sunflower, etc.

Soy products – tofu, tempeh, soy milk, etc.

Grains – quinoa, rice

Green superfoods – spirulina, Klamath Lake blue-green algae

Complete Protein

The only problem with plant sources of protein, with the exception of soybeans and quinoa, is that they aren't complete proteins because they don't provide all the amino acids. You should eat food combinations which form complete proteins, such as:

Legumes + seeds

Legumes + nuts

Legumes + dairy

Grains + legumes

Grains + dairy

Chances are you already eat complete proteins without even trying. Here are some tasty and healthy complete protein combinations:

- Cashew stir-fry with quinoa
- Beans on toast
- Cereal/muesli with milk
- Corn and beans
- Granola with yoghurt
- Hummus and pitta bread
- Nut butter with milk or wholegrain bread
- Three-bean chilli with cheese
- Rice and beans, peas or lentils
- Rice with milk (rice pudding)
- Split pea soup with wholegrain or seeded crackers or bread
- Tortillas with refried beans
- Veggie burgers with rice and peas

Make sure you guard against any nutrient deficiencies with fortified cereals, or have Marmite or Vegemite to get vitamin B_{12}. Try to eat a large portion of green leafy vegetables each day, and half a pint of skimmed or soy milk to ensure your calcium intake. Dried fruits, pulses, green veggies, dark chocolate and whole grains are good sources of iron, and choose butter fortified with vitamins D and E.

⇨ SAMPLE PROTEIN BOOST MENU
- *Breakfast:* Poached egg on granary toast
- *Mid-morning snack:* Cashews and raisins
- *Lunch:* Lean chicken or hummus, salad and crunchy vegetables (carrots,

lettuce, radish, peppers, broccoli, spring onions); sprinkling of toasted pine nuts

- *Mid-afternoon snack:* Glass of skimmed milk; apple
- *Dinner:* Tofu or seaweed stir fry with soy, ginger and vegetables (baby corn, mange tout, onions); berries and chocolate soya

9) ANTIOXIDANTS – ARE YOU GETTING ENOUGH?

We're on the home stretch now, and you should find the final two changes relatively easy. This is because if you've been following steps 1 to 8, chances are you'll already be doing them without realizing. But the health benefits for women with PCOS of these final two suggestions are so powerful that we've decided to highlight them.

Let's begin with antioxidants – a group of vitamins, minerals and unique compounds with special health benefits that are fantastic for women with PCOS.

WHY?

Our bodies are actually battlegrounds for infection and diseases. Simple body functions such as breathing or physical activity, and other lifestyle habits, such as smoking, produce substances called *free radicals* that attack healthy cells and arteries. Without intervention, free radicals wreak havoc at a cellular level and make you more susceptible to heart disease, certain types of cancers and signs of premature ageing (including wrinkles).

Antioxidants in your body work to counteract the action of free radicals, and for women with PCOS research[13] has shown them to be extremely beneficial for long-term health and daily vitality.

HOW?

Make sure you're getting plenty of antioxidants in your diet every day by eating lots of fruits, vegetables and wholegrains – ideally five portions of vegetables and three portions of fruit a day.

A vegetable portion is a mug-full of raw vegetables or a small cup of cooked. A fruit portion is one medium banana, orange or apple. (Remember, when you eat your fruit always have some protein at the same time, like some low-fat cheese or a handful of nuts.)

Fresh-pressed juices, smoothies, soups and frozen vegetables all count towards your portions, and you can maximize their antioxidant power by eating them raw. The next best thing is to steam or stir-fry rather than boil. If you must boil, keep the nutrient-rich water or stock to use in soups or casseroles.

Antioxidant Power

Beta Carotene: Beta carotene is one of 50 carotenoids in foods that convert to vitamin A in the body. It's usually found in red- and orange-coloured fruits and vegetables and in some dark green ones. Food sources include red, orange, deep-yellow and some dark-green leafy vegetables, carrots, sweet potatoes, broccoli, apricots, cantaloupe, mangoes, red and yellow peppers. You may also have heard of the carotenoid lycopene, found in tomatoes and which appears to protect against many diseases, including cancers.

Vitamin E: Helps protect the body from cell damage that can lead to cancer, heart disease, and cataracts as we age. Vitamin E works together with other antioxidants, such as vitamin C, to offer protection from diabetes and heart disease. Food sources include cold-pressed vegetable oils, wheat germ, wholegrain products, seeds, nuts and oily fish.

Vitamin C: The most famous antioxidant is vitamin C. Vitamin C is also known as ascorbic acid. Besides being an antioxidant, vitamin C plays an important role in fighting infections and keeping the walls of blood vessels firm, and gums healthy. Vitamin C is water soluble and is not retained in your body, so try to top up your levels every day with citrus fruits (oranges, grapefruits, tangerines), sweet peppers, strawberries, kiwis, broccoli and potato skins.

Selenium: If you eat a variety of grains from various places, you have a better chance of an adequate intake of the anti-cancer antioxidant selenium, but many countries have now got such poor levels of selenium in the soil that an increasing number of doctors worldwide recommend a supplement (one company in the UK has even launched a selenium-rich bread made from wheat grown on naturally enriched soil). Selenium is found in nuts, seafood, red meats, poultry, cereals, barley and other grains and breads.

Zinc: When zinc is deficient in the diet, metabolic rate drops and this can trigger blood sugar and hormone imbalances. Zinc is found in spinach, broccoli, green peas, green beans, tomato juice, lentils, oysters, shrimp, crab, turkey (dark meat), lean ham, lean ground beef, sunflower seeds, oily fish, lean sirloin steak, plain yoghurt, Swiss cheese, tofu and ricotta cheese.

⇨ SURPRISING SOURCES OF ANTIOXIDANTS

Red Wine: Two glasses of red wine a day provides a great source of antioxidants. More than this will have the opposite effect and leave you less, not more, able to fight off infections. Red wine contains bioflavenoids, which help towards reducing blood clots and, therefore, strokes. You need to drink three times the amount of blackcurrant juice to get the same effect as red wine – seven glasses of orange juice or 12 glasses of white wine.

Dark chocolate: Dark (not milk) chocolate provides one of the richest sources of antioxidants called catechins. Although good for you, chocolate in itself is still a fattening food, so eat it in moderation.

Brazil nuts: Brazils are very rich in selenium, and as little as three nuts a day will fulfil your requirements. Cashews, walnuts and almonds are nearly as good. Research has shown that when selenium levels are too low in the body, the risk of cancer is greatly increased.

Blueberries: There's evidence that natural antioxidant chemicals in fruit can reverse age-related memory loss. Blueberries and many richly coloured fruits such as strawberries – and veg like spinach – will help with this natural 'brain fix'.

Green tea: Green tea is a far healthier choice than black tea … although all are good at reducing the risk of heart disease by boosting the antioxidant action in blood plasma. A single cup of green tea a day brings great health benefits. Studies show that green tea drinkers are far less likely to develop hypertension – up to 46 per cent less in fact. People who drink more than four cups can cut hypertension by 65 per cent!

▷ **SAMPLE ANTIOXIDANT-RICH MENU**

- *Breakfast:* fruit salad, mixed seeds; glass of skimmed organic milk
- *Mid-morning snack:* Dried apricots or pear; 3 Brazil nuts
- *Lunch:* Vegetable and lentil soup; granary roll with cottage cheese and tomatoes or red peppers; apple tart with raspberries and soya cream
- *Mid-afternoon snack:* Grapes or cherries; 3 walnuts; 3 squares dark chocolate
- *Dinner:* Baked sweet potato with chickpea, tomato, peppers, onions, garlic topping; big green salad (spring onions, lettuce, cucumber, broccoli, green beans, avocado); steamed apple with cinnamon and raisins; small glass of red wine

10) EAT MORE PHYTOESTROGENS

Phytoestrogens are trace substances in our food which mimic and supplement the action of the body's own oestrogen. They are a comparatively recent discovery, and researchers are exploring the nutritional role of these substances in such diverse metabolic functions as the regulation of cholesterol and maintaining proper bone density post-menopause.

Phytoestrogens mainly fall into three classes:

1. Isoflavones – found in legumes such as lentils and soy beans
2. Lignans – found in nearly all grains and vegetables, the best source being linseeds
3. Coumestans – found mainly in alfalfa and mung bean sprouts.

WHY?

Phytoestrogens have a similar chemical structure to the oestrogen your body produces, and this may explain their hormone-balancing effect. Studies[14] show that they not only can take the place of natural oestrogens and increase oestrogen levels when they are too low, they can also reduce them when they are too high, by fastening on to your body's oestrogen receptors and giving off a weaker signal than your own body's oestrogen molecules would. As well as helping to balance hormones, phytoestrogens are also thought to have a protective effect on the heart. Studies[15] show they can lower levels of bad (LDL) cholesterol. It's also thought they may contain compounds that can inhibit breast and endometrial cancer (often due to excess oestrogen) and protect from osteoporosis.

HOW?

According to UK nutritionist Dr Marilyn Glenville, the recommended amount is about 45mg of isoflavones a day. So how do you reach your 45mg?

Vegetables, in particular green leafy or cruciferous vegetables such as broccoli, cabbage and Brussels sprouts (which have been shown to have hormone-balancing and anti-cancer properties[16]) are a great source of phytoestrogens. Legumes are another good source. Soya, lentils, beans and chickpeas contain phytoestrogens in the form of isoflavones. An 8oz serving of soyamilk contains approximately 25mg of isoflavones. Half a cup of soy beans, tofu or tempeh contains approximately 40mg of isoflavones. At present the recommended amount to ensure 45mg is one serving of soyfood with plenty of wholegrains, fruits and vegetables and legumes a day.

There has been some concern about the aluminium levels in soya, which have been linked to Alzheimer's, but eaten in moderation – say two or three times a week – soya can be good for women with PCOS as studies have shown that in small amounts it can reduce cholesterol levels. Don't eat too much, though, as preliminary research also suggests that large quantities of soya may increase the risk of heart disease. The best way to eat soya is in its traditional form, choosing products such as miso, tofu or organic soya, and to avoid snack bars made from processed soy beans.

Other sources of phytoestrogen include cinnamon, sage, red clover, hops, fennel and parsley, all fruits (especially apples, plums, cherries, cranberries, blueberries and citrus fruits), whole grains such as rice, oats, barley, rye and wheat, and seeds including linseeds, sesame, pumpkin, poppy, caraway and sunflower.

⇨ SIX GOLDEN RULES

1. Eat at least five portions of vegetables and three portions of fruit a day.
2. Eat more nutritious foods and eat them often.
3. Cut down on the Ss: salt, sugar and saturated fat, and increase the Fs: fluids, fish and fibre.
4. Every day, aim for around 50 per cent carbohydrates (whole food and low GI, of course) 20 to 25 per cent healthy fat, and 20 to 25 per cent good-quality protein.
5. Remember the 80/20 rule. If you eat well 80 per cent of the time, you can splurge the other 20 without worry.
6. Enjoy all kinds of food in moderation and enjoy experimenting with new flavours.

PCOS FRIENDLY MEAL IDEAS

BREAKFASTS

- Bowl of porridge, hot oat cereal or muesli. Serve with semi-skimmed, skimmed or soy milk. Add fresh and dried fruit if needed instead of sugar.
- Two slices of granary/multigrain toast with a smidge of spreadable butter.
- One slice of granary/multigrain toast topped with any of the following: 1 egg, half a tin of reduced-salt baked beans, tinned fish without extra oil, extra light soft cheese.
- Two portions of fruit with low-calorie yoghurt.

LUNCHES

- Sandwiches made with granary/multigrain/rye bread or pitta. Low-fat spread on bread and any low-fat filling such as:
Tuna (in brine) with cucumber (use low-fat mayonnaise/salad cream if required); Salmon and cucumber; Ham and tomato; Chicken/turkey and salad; Reduced fat hummus with raw spinach, rocket or salad; Cottage cheese or extra light soft cheese with salad.
- Salads based on wholewheat pasta or basmati rice, such as:
Pasta with tuna, sweetcorn and chopped peppers mixed with low-fat dressing; Pasta with tinned salmon and low-fat dressing served with salad; Pasta in tomato sauce served with salad; Basmati rice with chicken, chopped raw onion and a few flaked almonds dressed with a little low-fat mayonnaise, mild curry powder and a teaspoon of chutney, served with a large salad.

- Jacket potato (medium) with cottage cheese and pineapple or tomatoes; baked beans and low-fat cheese; tuna and low-fat mayonnaise or cottage cheese – all served with a big green salad.
- Soups – try chunky vegetable; carrot and corriander; Tuscan bean; or fresh tomato and basil with seeds sprinkled on top, and a wholegrain roll with cottage cheese or lean chicken.

DINNER

Serve all these with a colourful, crunchy side salad or steamed vegetables.

- Wholegrain pasta with a tomato or pesto sauce. Add tuna, chicken or a little grated mature cheese.
- Vegetable curry (e.g. chickpeas and vegetables with low-fat sauce) served with boiled brown basmati rice.
- Spaghetti bolognese (make sure you use lean mince or quorn, and drain off the fat before adding the sauce).
- Meat or tofu curry: Stir-fry lean meat in a little pure vegetable oil with onions. Add any other vegetables and stir in a low-fat cooking sauce. Serve with boiled basmati rice, topped with seeds.
- Reduced-salt baked beans on granary/multigrain toast.
- Salmon steak grilled or cooked and served with new potatoes and vegetables or salad. Try serving with a teaspoon of dill and mustard sauce.
- Mackerel, pilchards or sardines (tinned in brine or tomato sauce) with granary toast.
- Chunky vegetable and pulse (e.g. chickpeas, lentils, butterbeans) casserole.

- Tofu/Soya sausages, with a small serving of mashed potato.
- Wholegrain pitta stuffed with grilled slices of halloumi cheese and lean chicken or turkey.
- Omelette (2 eggs) packed with herbs (e.g. basil, mint and chives).
- Wholegrain bread (2 slices) topped with tomato paste, fresh vegetables and low-fat hard cheese – grill to make healthy pizzas.

DESSERTS

- Fruit or low-fat, low-sugar yoghurt.
- Fruit (the less ripe the better, as the riper the fruit the higher the GI).
- Oat-based cereal bars (though some can be high in fat and sugar).
- A bowl of skimmed milk custard or rice pudding with chopped fruit.
- A big fruit salad with 6 chunks of melted dark chocolate as a sauce.
- Fruit tart with raspberries.
- Baked apples stuffed with raisins and cinnamon with soya cream.
- Grilled peach halves or pears with a sprinkle of brown sugar.

For chocolate cravings try low-calorie hot chocolate without sweeteners or soya hot chocolate, a light chocolate mousse or a few squares of quality dark chocolate.

DRINKS

- Sugar-free or no-added-sugar squash
- Tea or coffee without milk
- Fruit and veggie juices and smoothies
- Filtered water

Select drinks that are low in both alcohol and sugar – for example, light beer and dry wine are good choices. Use diet soft drinks or water to mix drinks and don't forget to limit yourself to no more than five or six alcoholic drinks a week.

CHAPTER 7
EXERCISE –YOUR PCOS-BEATING PLAN

Physical activity is an essential key to managing PCOS – it improves insulin resistance in people who are obese or have diabetes, helps maintain a healthy weight, lifts your mood, protects your heart, cuts your risk of diabetes, high blood pressure and certain cancers such as breast cancer, reduces stress and improves your self-esteem and energy levels.

AND IF YOU'VE GOT PCOS ...

A number of studies have demonstrated that exercise can do fabulous things for your health.

A study[1] conducted at the University of Adelaide in Australia showed that a six-month programme of diet and exercise helped 18 overweight PCOS women normalize their hormones. They experienced an 11 per cent reduction in central fat (around their stomachs), 71 per cent improvement in insulin sensitivity, 33 per cent fall in insulin levels, and a 39 per cent reduction in LH (luteinizing hormone) levels. This study is relevant because insulin resistance and chronically high insulin and LH levels are reasons why women with PCOS don't ovulate and why they have a number of other troubling symptoms.

Exercise can help you normalize your insulin metabolism, which in turn will reduce your testosterone levels and all the PCOS symptoms associated with this – acne, excess hair, weight gain and irregular periods.

Regular exercise can also help control your PCOS symptoms because it helps you to lose weight by reducing insulin resistance – and this links in to the 'apple' and 'pear' body-shape health risks mentioned earlier. For most women, carrying extra weight around their waists or middle (with a waist larger than 35 inches) increases health risks (like heart disease, diabetes, or cancer) more than carrying extra weight around their hips or thighs.

⇨ APPLE OR PEAR?

Get your tape measure out and measure your waist and hips. If your waist number is higher than your hip number, you're an apple. If your hips are wider than your waist, you're a pear.

Now divide your waist measurement by your hip measurement. Women with a waist-to-hip ratio greater than 0.8 are at greater risk of diabetes, high blood pressure and heart disease.

According to a study[2] from Syracuse University in New York, exercise is necessary for the loss of belly fat in women with diabetes. Thirty-three women were divided into 'diet only' and 'diet plus exercise' groups. Since women with diabetes have metabolic problems similar to those of women with PCOS, the study results are relevant. Either diet alone, or diet plus exercise, caused an average weight loss of 9.9 lb in three months. But only the diet-plus-exercise group had a loss of visceral fat, which is the belly fat that surrounds internal organs.

Another study[3] at the University of Warwick in England has provided the first evidence that regular exercise significantly lowers homocysteine levels in the blood and reduces belly fat in overweight women with PCOS. In this study, a group of women who exercised for six months had a significant drop in their homocysteine levels. They also reduced their waist-to-hip ratio. In contrast, there was no change in the non-exercising group.

And this counts for moderate exercise as well – research shows that low to moderate exercise may actually be better for women with PCOS than high-intensity exercise.[4]

Regular exercise also speeds up your metabolism and balances your hormones. Studies show that fit people burn more calories even when they are at rest. It takes more calories to maintain muscle tissue than fat tissue. So the more you exercise the more your muscles build up and the speedier your metabolism becomes.

With research[5] continuing to confirm that regular, moderate exercise can lower blood sugar levels, promote insulin efficiency, lower blood pressure and the risk of a heart attack and diabetes, keeping fit may be one of the most effective ways for you to control your symptoms, prevent any need for medication, boost your self-esteem and, of course, lose weight.

HOW MUCH?

Our bodies were made to move. For centuries we were nomads travelling in search of food. Once we learned how to create our food supply, we were able to stay in one place. As time passed and technology advanced, our lives became more and more sedentary. Today the majority of us find ourselves with a lifestyle that actually demands very little movement or effort. Our bodies, however, are still hard-wired for movement, and not using them causes untold health issues.

To manage your symptoms and lower the long-term health risks associated with PCOS, all you need is 30 minutes of moderate-intensity physical activity, above your usual activity, at work or home on most days of the week. If you can't set aside one block of time, or your fitness levels aren't there yet, try short bursts of activity such as three 10-minute walks. If you can do more, go for it and extend your daily workout to 60 minutes. Don't overdo it, though, as research shows that over-exercising can have a negative effect on your health and well-being. Always consult your doctor before starting a new exercise plan, particularly if you:

- have heart disease or have had a stroke or are at high risk for them
- have diabetes or are at high risk for it
- are overweight or obese
- have an injury (like a knee injury)
- are over 50
- are pregnant.

On top of your exercise session, try to boost your exercise further by increasing activity levels in your daily life. Get off the bus a few stops earlier and walk, take the stairs instead of the lift, walk to the shops, and so on. When it comes to exercise, every little helps.

YOUR DAILY ROUTINE

Once you've made the decision to exercise regularly the next thing you need to know is what exercise goals you should be setting. A good exercise routine that you can repeat daily or three to five times a week at least starts with 5 to 10 minutes of gentle warm up, such as walking at a moderate pace, to raise your body temperature and increase your heart rate.

WARM-UP EXERCISES

Try the following exercises (at least three to five repetitions each) for a warm-up routine:

Forward Arm Reach: Position arms out front, palms facing one another. Raise one or both arms as high as possible (one arm may help the other if needed). Slowly lower to starting position.

Shoulder Shrug: Stand erect. Raise one or both shoulders up towards your ears. Lower and repeat.

Neck: Slowly turn your neck to the right and hold for a count of 2. Then turn it to the left and hold for a count of 2. Tilt your head forward for a count of 2 and upward for a count of 2. Repeat.

Side Leg Lift: Stand straight, with a chair at your left side to hold on to for balance. Lift your right leg up and out to the side. Then cross that leg in front of the other leg. Turn round and repeat with your left leg.

Spine: Keeping your arms straight, reach up with both arms, hold for 5 seconds and lower. Place your hands on your hips and slowly tilt your upper body to the left and hold for a count of 2. Return to centre and repeat to the right, holding for a count of 2. Repeat.

Hips and knees: With your body upright, move your hips by bending and lifting your left knee as far as is comfortable. Hold for a count of 2, then lower. Now raise your right knees and hold to a count of 2. Lower. Repeat.

Pulse-raising: Walking is a good way to elevate your temperature, increase your blood flow and prepare your body for exercise. It can also get you energized for more strenuous exercise. If weather permits, walk to the end of your driveway or street and back. Walk around your house one or more times. Walk or march in place for several minutes. For weight loss you need to get your heart rate up to 60 to 75 per cent of its maximum capacity (220 minus your age) for around 20 to 45 minutes. If you feel slightly out of breath but not so much that you can't carry on a conversation, you know you are exercising at the right rate. A cool-down should follow your aerobic workout.

AEROBIC EXERCISES

After your warm-up you'll be ready for a period of continuous moderately paced aerobic conditioning. Aim for 20 to 30 minutes of continuous exercise that works the large muscles of the body and elevates your breathing and heart rate. Fast walking is ideal, or you may prefer jogging, swimming or an exercise class.

For weight loss you need to get your heart rate up to 60 to 75 per cent of its maximum capacity (220 minus your age) for around 20 to 45 minutes. If you feel slightly out of breath but not so much that you can't carry on a conversation, you know you're exercising at the right rate.

The following aerobic exercises are great for women with PCOS.

Walking: When you first begin your walking programme, start slowly, maybe trying a 5-minute stroll. Each time you walk, increase your intensity by walking faster and for longer until you're walking for 20 or 30 minutes. You can also add light handweights. If you don't want to walk outside you may want to use a treadmill.

Swimming: Swimming is a great way to exercise as it works every muscle in the body with the minimum of stress. Start by going to the pool twice a week for a gentle 15-minute swim. Gradually increase the length of your swim and your work rate while in the water. Aim to build up to about 30 minutes a day, or 45 minutes twice a week. You might also want to try some aquarobics classes.

Cycling / cycle-machine, or Jogging: Start with a short easy routine of 10–15 minutes per day, gradually working up to about 30 minutes a day. Gradually increase your work rate, without ever straining yourself. If jogging, please invest in a good pair of running shoes that offer cushioned support.

Trampoline jogging: You can buy small, inexpensive trampolines from most sports shops. Gently jogging on a small trampoline can be a good aerobic workout. Try to keep going for 20 to 30 minutes.

Dancing: You can join a class, go to a disco or just boogie away at home. Dancing isn't just fun, it's a great way to exercise and release tension.

STRETCHING EXERCISES

You need also to have a daily routine that stretches your muscles and puts your joints through their full range of motion. The best time to stretch is when your muscles are warmed up after your aerobic workout. Allow about 10 minutes for stretching. Stretching your muscles keeps you flexible. It also lengthens your muscles and improves posture.

Stretching exercises can also be done on their own, first thing in the morning and last thing at night.

A good stretch needs to be held for 20–30 seconds for each muscle group. Try the stretches without any bouncy movements, and as you do them keep breathing rhythmic, slow and under control. For example, if you're doing forward bends, inhale while coming forward, breathe slowly during the stretch and exhale while coming up. Do not hold your breath during stretching exercises.

Shoulder Stretch: Stand with your feet slightly apart. Raise your right arm. Bending at the elbow, bring your right arm across your chest at shoulder level until you feel a slight pull in your shoulder. Gently apply pressure with your left hand at your right elbow. Stay in this position for a few seconds, then relax. Repeat with your left arm.

Chest Stretch: Stand just outside an open doorway (the doorway should be behind you) and face outward. Grab both sides of the doorframe at chest level. Take a step forward and let your arms straighten behind you. Keep your head up and lean forward until you feel a stretch in your chest muscles. Stay in this position for a few seconds, then relax.

Another method is to hold your arms out behind you, keeping your knees slightly bent and your pelvis tucked under. Move your shoulders and elbows back until you feel a gentle stretch.

Back Arch: Stand with your feet slightly apart and knees slightly bent. Place your hands on the front of your thighs and bend forward slightly at the waist, without curving your back. Slowly inhale and arch your back. Stay in this position for a few seconds, then exhale. Straighten and return to the standing position. Repeat.

You could also stand with your feet slightly apart and knees slightly bent. Place your hands on your hips and lean slightly back. Be sure not to lean too far back! Stay in this position for a few seconds, then relax. Repeat.

Calf Stretches: Stand facing a wall, with your feet about three feet away from the wall. Place your hands on the wall at about shoulder level. Keeping your feet flat on the floor, lean forward until you feel a slight stretch in your calves. Stay in this position for a few seconds, then relax. Repeat.

Another stretching exercise for the calves is to raise both heels off the floor so you're on your toes. Repeat 10 times. As your calf muscles strengthen you should be able to stay on your toes for longer periods of time.

Front Thigh Stretch: Stand facing a wall, with your feet about three feet from the wall. Place your right hand on the wall at chest level. Bend your left leg backwards. Use your left hand to grab the top of your left foot behind you. Gently pull your heel towards your buttocks. Stay in this position for a few seconds, then relax. Repeat with your right leg.

Groin: Stand with your feet slightly apart, your hips forward and your back straight. Bend your left leg to one side while moving your right leg slowly the other way, keeping it straight until you feel a gentle stretch in your groin. Gently move to the right, bending your right leg as you straighten the left.

MUSCLE STRENGTH

You also need to include some muscle strengthening activities into your routine around two or three times a week – building up better muscle tone not only makes you look more streamlined but also boosts your metabolism so you burn more calories even when you're not exercising.

Walking and cycling are good weight-bearing endurance exercises, but strength training is even better. The aim is not to become muscle bound – you need only do a few sets of exercises such as press ups and squats. Fitness clubs offer weights and weight machines, but if you can't face the gym you can get some benefits working out at home with some light dumbbells or heavy books/tins or water bottles. An exercise video can also help. To get the most out of weight training, you need to take the time to learn the correct technique.

Try to exercise two or three times a week, working all your different muscles. Repeat each exercise 10 to 15 times (a set) and do one or two sets of each exercise.

Upper body: Push-ups will strengthen your shoulders, arms and chest. Balance the weight between your hands, which should be placed directly beneath your shoulders. Keeping your back straight, gradually lower your chest so that it nearly touches the floor, bending your elbows. Return to the starting position – without locking your elbows. If you wish to concentrate on strengthening your arm muscles, move your hands closer together.

For the upper back, lie face-down on the floor and, keeping your legs straight, gently raise your head and shoulders. Hold for a count of 2 and then lower.

Middle body: Lie flat on your back on the floor and bring your knees up to about a 90-degree angle. Then, with your hands positioned either behind your head (do not pull on your neck as you come up) or reaching forward, slowly lift your upper body using your abdominal muscles. Keep your back rounded throughout the movement – it's very important not to arch it.

Concentrate on pushing your lower back into the floor. You can vary the exercise by reaching forward to the right or left of your raised legs; this will use slightly different muscles. You can alternate from side to side or do 5 on one side, then 5 on the other, or whatever you can comfortably manage.

Lower body: Lie on your back and lift your right leg, pulling it towards your chest until you feel a gentle pull in your bottom and lower back. Repeat with the left leg. Now pull both legs up together.

'Sit' with your back against a wall so your knees are bent. Hold the position for as long as you can. This may only be around 10 seconds to start off with, but you should be able to build up to a minute.

Working with weights: You can use some light dumbbells, but if you haven't got these a bag of sugar or a tin of baked beans will do.

From a seated or standing position, hold the weights just above your shoulders. Push them up overhead slowly.

Making sure your upper body moves, turn to the left, swinging both arms as you turn. Repeat 10 times. Now perform the same exercise swinging your body and arms to the right.

COOLING DOWN

Always finish your workout by cooling down, using the warm-up exercises and stretching exercises on pages 105–6 and 108–9.

HOW CAN I PREVENT INJURY WHEN I EXERCISE?

If you haven't been very active for some time or have a medical problem, start your programme with short sessions (5 to 10 minutes) of physical activity and build up to your goal. Before you start, be sure to warm up for 5 to 10 minutes. Use the right equipment –whether it's walking shoes, running shoes or knee pads – and make sure it's in good condition and right for your skill level. Drink water before, during and after exercise. If your chest feels tight or painful, or you feel faint or have trouble breathing at any time, stop the activity straight away and talk to your doctor or health-care provider.

⇨ TONE UP YOUR TUMMY

As we tend to gain weight around the waist, the following tips will help trim those tums:

1. Aerobic workouts increase your metabolism for up to 24 hours or more! This means you're less likely to store any excess calories, plus you're more likely to burn off excess body fat in the process!
2. Combine regular aerobic exercises with toning exercises such as this one:

Basic Crunch

Lie flat on your back with your knees bent and feet flat on the floor. Place your hands lightly behind your head for support. Using your abdominal muscles lift your shoulders a few inches off the ground, pause briefly and return to your starting position. Complete at least one set of 10–12 reps. Rest for a minute, then repeat.

The crunch is the single best exercise for toning the abdominal wall. However, to flatten the stomach you need to do The Plank.

The Plank

Lie flat on your stomach and place your hands on either side of your chest – as if ready to perform a press-up – although you should tuck your elbows into your sides. Keeping your back perfectly flat, push yourself up onto your knees – so that your upper body is off the floor, with your hands and knees acting as support. Keeping your back flat, pull in your tummy button as high as possible – as if to suck it in close to your spine. Aim to maintain a normal breathing pattern and hold this position for 10–60 seconds. Rest, lie flat, then repeat twice.

1. Watch your posture. Poor posture or slumping as you walk can make even a flat tum look saggy. Good posture has nothing to do with the old-school regime of pulling in your stomach and puffing your chest out. Good posture is about keeping your body upright and stomach firm by using the muscles that run along your back and spine and legs to lift you up.
2. If bloating is making your stomach look flabby, take a look at our 'beat the bloat' tips on page 231.
3. Any alcoholic drinks can add to the size of your stomach because they cause bloating and are dense in calories. If you can't give up completely,

bear in mind that beer drinkers tend to have the highest waist-to-hip-ratios, while wine drinkers have the slimmest waistlines.

4. If you feel you need an extra boost, enlist the help of a professional trainer. You don't need to go for a regular weekly slot; one or two sessions should be enough to teach you some basics. A qualified fitness trainer can help you achieve your health and fitness goals, and in less time than you might imagine. If gyms and personal trainers aren't your scene, buy a book or video with plenty of advice about toning the stomach area.

WHAT IF I'M OVERWEIGHT?

Very large people face special challenges trying to be active. You may not be able to bend or move in the same way other people do. It may be hard to find clothes and equipment for exercising. You may feel self-conscious being active around other people.

Facing these challenges is hard, but it can be done! Non-weight-bearing activities, like swimming or water workouts, put less stress on your joints because you don't have to lift or push your own weight. And if you can't do something, don't be hard on yourself. Pat yourself on the back for trying even if you can't do something first time. It may be easier the next time – so try again! Just moving any part of your body – even for a short time – makes you healthier.

WHAT IF I'M TOO TIRED?

Studies[6] have shown that people who exercise regularly (as long as they aren't exercising just before they go to sleep) fall asleep more quickly and spend more of the night in deep sleep than their sedentary peers. These benefits are found in people of all ages, even older adults who, as a group, tend to experience more problems with sleep and fatigue. In one study, older adults who began exercising four times a week reported falling asleep 15 minutes faster and sleeping about an hour longer than at the beginning of the 16-week study.

In short, the less you exercise the more tired you are going to feel. Try to exercise even if you feel tired. If you think you're too tired at night, plan to exercise in the morning. You will have more energy as soon as you start moving. Listening to music can also help motivate you. It's true — exercise actually gives you more energy in the long run!

SOME TIPS TO GET YOU GOING

Getting started with an exercise routine can be tough. We hope the following tips will help get you going.

- Choose an activity that's fun. Find an activity you enjoy, so you can maintain a positive attitude. This can include dancing, horse-riding, rambling, etc. — it doesn't have to be a traditional form of exercise.
- Change your activities and exercise routine, so you don't get bored.

- Doing housework may not be fun, but it does get you moving! So does gardening, yard work and walking the dog.
- If you can't set aside one block of time, do short activities during the day, such as three 10-minute walks.
- Create opportunities for activity, such as parking your car a few streets away from where you need to be, taking the stairs instead of the lift, or walking down the hall to talk to a co-worker instead of using e-mail.
- Don't let the cold weather keep you on the couch! You can still find activities to do in the winter, like exercising to a workout video or joining a sports league. Or get a headstart on your spring cleaning by washing the windows or re-organizing your cupboards.
- Use different jogging, walking, or biking paths to vary your routine.
- Exercise with a friend or family member. It's tougher to break the commitment to exercise when you know someone else will be working out with you.
- If you have children, make time to play with them outside. Set a positive example!
- Make activities into social occasions – have dinner after you and a friend work out.
- Read fitness books or magazines to inspire you.
- Set specific short-term fitness goals, and reward yourself when you achieve them.
- Don't feel bad if you don't notice body changes straight away.
- Make your activity a regular part of your day, so it becomes a habit.
- Team up with some other women who've got PCOS to organize walking clubs, exercise classes or special events such as a disco or charity fun run to promote physical activity.

STILL NEED MOTIVATION?

If you still feel reluctant to exercise on a regular basis, consider this: In addition to unpleasant day-to-day symptoms such as acne, irregular periods and weight gain, PCOS puts you at considerable risk of a host of serious health problems including diabetes, heart disease and obesity – and an exercise programme, even one as simple as walking 15 to 30 minutes a day – can significantly reduce not just the day-to-day symptoms but also your risk of poor health in the future.

Making exercise a regular part of your life is a powerful path towards a healthier, happier and longer life, managing your symptoms and maintaining healthy body weight. Taking time out of your day for walking, cycling or taking an exercise class could add years – healthy, energetic years – to your future.

CHAPTER 8
YOUR HEALTH-BOOSTING LIFESTYLE DETOX

In our day-to-day lives it's estimated[1] that there are now hundreds of chemicals that didn't exist 60 years ago that deplete nutrients, collect in our bodies and interfere with hormonal health.

Every day a sea of potentially hormone-disturbing toxins surrounds us: environmental solvents, plastics and adhesives, toxins in make up, nail polish, hair dyes and shampoos as well as household cleaners. The air we breathe contains pollutants from car exhausts and cigarette smoke. Even food and soil are inundated with pesticides, not forgetting the chemicals and additives in processed foods.

The uncomfortable truth is, more and more research[2] suggests that these chemicals are threatening our health with a new kind of pollution that contaminates our bodies.

HORMONE-DISRUPTING CHEMICALS

Government spokespeople will tell us that hormonally active agents or HAA (chemicals in the environment that mimic our own natural hormones) – also known as petrochemicals, xeno-oestrogens or endocrine-disrupting chemicals (EDCs) – are safe. They're found in everything from plastics to pesticides and, of course, the residues of hormonal medications that don't break down once they pass into our water supply. Preliminary research[3] reports on their potentially damaging effects to our hormonal and general health.

Research[4] in 2002 from Brunel University reported on a five-year study which found sex changes in male fish in UK rivers contaminated with synthetic (man-made) oestrogens. Scientists blame the pollution on a 'potent' form of oestrogen found in urine from women using the contraceptive pill, flushed through sewage works and into rivers. Dr Susan Joblin has been quoted as saying, 'One could argue that we are living in a sea of oestrogen, a chemical cocktail, and therefore I think there are real reasons to be worried about health and fertility.'

EVERYDAY TOXINS

Other studies show that everyday substances such as cigarettes, alcohol and coffee can contain toxins that upset our hormones and increase the risk of infertility and even cancer. Women exposed to heavy metals and chemicals such as lead, aluminium and cadmium are also more likely to have irregular periods and experience fertility problems.[5]

It makes sense, in this chemical world, if you have PCOS and want to give your body a helping hand to better health, to detox your lifestyle however you can.

DETOXING YOUR LIFE

You don't need to go on fasts, retreats or harsh health regimes to detox. What we mean by detox is trying to avoid unnecessary chemicals and pollutants that clog your system and make it harder for your body to work efficiently.

YOUR BODY'S IN-HOUSE DETOX SYSTEM

All day, every day, your liver, kidneys and adrenal glands work to keep your hormones functioning efficiently and you feeling healthy and vital. These organs are crucial for the removal of potentially harmful toxins which can disrupt hormonal systems and trigger the symptoms of PCOS.

THE LIVER

Your liver is a chemical clearing house. Every minute of the day it cleans one-and-a-half quarts of blood so that other organs can be nourished with purified blood. It also neutralizes toxic wastes, sending them off to the kidneys for elimination. The liver also removes excess hormones such as oestrogens, thereby maintaining hormonal balance. In addition, it produces amino acids and enzymes to metabolize fat, proteins and carbs, and helps regulate blood sugar levels.

Drugs, alcohol, fatty foods, smoking and other environmental toxins, from pesticides and exhaust fumes to hairsprays, can overload the liver. If the liver is overloaded it will force your other detoxifying organs (skin, lymph, kidneys, adrenals) to work overtime, which can cause rashes, acne, testosterone excess, bloating, yeast infections and poor health.

THE KIDNEYS

Your kidneys work alongside your liver to eliminate waste from your body. Your kidneys help maintain mineral balance and they also pull out unwanted elements like chemicals. When the filtering is complete, urine flows from the kidneys to the bladder. If your liver is overloaded with toxins and chemicals, the excess passes to your kidneys. Trouble is, your kidneys were not designed to detoxify waste, and so the toxins move to your urinary tract where they can cause infection.

ADRENAL GLANDS

Your adrenal glands manufacture hormones such as adrenaline and cortisol to help you cope with the stresses of everyday life. The more your adrenal glands are under siege because of physical, emotional or environmental stress, the greater the likelihood of adrenal exhaustion. When this happens too much cortisol is produced, which in turn can trigger testosterone production and symptoms of PCOS.

THE LYMPHATIC SYSTEM

Your lymph system is also crucial to your body's detox processes. Lymph, a liquid produced by the lymph glands in various parts of the body from your neck and armpits to your groin, absorbs dead cells, excess fluids and other waste products from food and takes them into the lymph nodes, where they are stored and eventually fed into the blood and on to one of eliminatory organs to be passed our via sweat, faeces or urine. Poor lymph drainage due to excess waste results in a build-up of toxins.

There are two important things you can do to help keep your liver, kidneys, adrenals and lymph system in good working order and protect yourself from toxins:

1. Give them the nutritional support they need. Nutrients can help process, transform or eliminate toxins and excess hormones. Follow the guidelines in Chapter 6 and make extra sure you're getting plenty of antioxidants (see page 90 for more information about antioxidants and how to make sure you include them in your diet).

2. Reduce the amount of toxins you're exposed to, in order to allow your body's natural detox systems to function properly. The 9-step PCOS detox plan that follows is designed to help you do just that.

9-STEP PCOS DETOX PLAN

1. IF YOU SMOKE, STOP

A report published in 2000 by then-UK Health Secretary Allan Milburn revealed that over 600 chemicals are allowed into cigarettes, some of which sound simply bizarre, like the radioactive material polonium acetone (also used to make paint-stripper) and ammonia (used in toilet cleaners).

Smoking damages almost all aspects of hormonal, sexual and reproductive health, according to a February 2004 report by the British Medical Association. It's a significant anti-nutrient and reduces the level of vitamin C in the bloodstream. Smokers also have high levels of cadmium, a heavy toxic metal that can keep the body from using zinc efficiently – and zinc is needed for a healthy menstrual cycle. Cigarettes cut down the number of fertile years a woman has to conceive, cause irregular periods and make eggs and cervical mucus less hospitable to sperm. In short, the more you smoke the more likely you are to have irregular periods and problems conceiving.

Smoking is one of the major causes of preventable disease, and if you've got PCOS doctors strongly advise against it.[6] Smoking drains oestrogen levels, and this can increase the risk of early menopause and conditions linked to lower oestrogen levels such as osteoporosis – and that's regardless of whether you smoke five or 20 cigarettes a day. Other studies link smoking with an increased risk of heart disease and breast and lung cancer.

Health risks increase dramatically if you're a smoker and are on the Pill, because both leach the nutrients you need to beat the symptoms of PCOS.

Quitting isn't easy, but here are some helpful tips:

- Researchers at the University of Pittsburgh School of Medicine found that women who quit smoking between the first and 14th day of their menstrual cycle had fewer withdrawal symptoms such as depression, anxiety or irritability.
- It's estimated that up to 304,000 people successfully quit smoking every year with the help of over-the-counter products such as nicotine gums and patches.

- Get counselling. Aim for four to seven sessions over a two-month period with a counsellor who is used to treating addictive conditions.
- Many women say that acupuncture can be extremely helpful with withdrawal symptoms.
- Hypnotherapy works by suggesting to your subconscious mind that you won't crave cigarettes.
- Many people say that gradually reducing the amount of cigarettes you smoke a day isn't helpful. You may find that the best way is to go cold turkey. The nicotine will pass out of your system after 48 hours, so you won't be craving that. What you'll be craving is the *habit* of smoking, for example using smoking as a time-out or as something to do with your hands. You need to replace the smoking habit with a more positive one. If you feel like you want a cigarette, go for a walk. If you don't know what to do with your hands, buy some worry beads. If you crave a smoke after a meal, pop a stick of chewing gum into your mouth.

You can help your liver and lungs recover from years of having smoked by supporting them with the nutrients they need to thrive. The nutritional strategy for smokers is to increase their intake of whole grains, raw seeds, nuts, legumes and fruits and vegetables and decrease their intake of fats, food additives and alcohol. Since smoking generates an acidic condition in the body, a whole-meal high-fibre diet helps by maintaining healthy bowel function. Research at St George's Hospital Medical School, London, published in the medical journal *Thorax* (January, 2000), has found that certain foods such as apples can boost lung health and healing. Organic unfiltered raw apple cider vinegar is a natural tonic for overall health, especially respiratory health. Dilute with water and drink a glass every day. Water is essential to balance out the drying effects of smoking.

Smoking leaches essential nutrients, so a general multivitamin with additional vitamin A, C, E and selenium is an important part of any smoker's quitting programme. The cadmium won't leave your body when you stop smoking; it needs to be tackled by supplementing your diet with these antioxidant supplements.

2. CUT DOWN ON CAFFEINE

Whether you're drinking coffee, tea, caffeinated soft drinks or even chocolate, low doses of caffeine can typically make you feel more alert and energetic. At higher doses, though, they can leave us feeling anxious, irritable and unable to switch off or sleep.

Over time too much caffeine weakens the adrenal glands, depletes vital nutrients and interferes with hormonal balance.[7] Caffeine has also been linked to irregular periods and infertility.[8] A cycle develops where greater and greater amounts are needed to achieve the familiar 'high', and symptoms such as headaches and indigestion can occur if we don't get our fix. In short, we're addicted.

So does all this mean we need to give up caffeine altogether if we have PCOS? Not completely. In general the weight of scientific evidence seems to suggest that a moderate amount of tea and coffee is OK and won't damage your health. Studies show, for example, that one or two cups of tea a day may cut your risk of heart disease because tea contains substances called catchins which are thought to protect against heart disease. Other studies suggest that one or two cups of coffee a day can help boost memory function in old age, and may even prevent diabetes.[9] It's excess that is dangerous. If you're drinking more than three cups of tea, coffee or caffeinated drinks a day, you need to cut down.

CAFFEINE CUT-BACK PLAN

- Make one cup of tea at a time instead of a whole pot.
- Buy a dainty cup and get rid of your jumbo-size mug.
- If you're at a coffee shop, always order a small rather than large one.
- Cut back gradually over a two- to three-week period. Lower your intake by drinking grain coffee blends or diluted or smaller amounts of regular coffee.
- Consider trying herbal coffee – available at health food stores or the health food section at your supermarket.
- Start cutting back during the weekend or on holiday when you're less busy and stressed.
- Choose caffeine-free soft drinks.
- Drink more water, fruit juice, vegetable juices and herbal teas. To save calories, dilute fruit juice with sparkling water or soda water.
- Experiment with herbal teas. We recommend roasted herbal roots such as barley, chicory and dandelion as coffee substitutes and teas such as lemon grass, peppermint, ginger-root, red clover, rosehip, apple, hibiscus, clover flower, nettles and chamomile.

3. FRESH, HEALTHY FOODS

Eating as much fresh (preferably raw) food as you can is important because these foods boost nutritional support to your body's detox system. It's also a good way to increases your intake of cleansing fibre, which not only encourages elimination but also prevents the absorption of oestrogen chemicals into your bloodstream. And the more fresh food you eat, the less likely you are to eat refined ones, which are often loaded with unwanted, hidden toxins and chemicals.

If you've been following the guidelines for a healthy PCOS diet you should already be eating plenty of fresh healthy food and avoiding refined foods and foods high in sugar and fat.

There's detox power in fresh food, especially if it's raw or as close to its natural state as possible. Raw food is loaded with nutrient enzymes. Vital to life, enzymes work tirelessly at breaking down food, assisting the digestive system, boosting immune system, carrying on the functions of metabolism and removing toxins from the body.

We are not saying you should always eat fresh, raw food – our digestive systems can't take that – but we are saying it's important to eat plenty of it. Here are some easy ways to incorporate more fresh foods into your diet:

- Soups and salads made from fresh vegetables, grains and legumes are easy to make and keep.
- Use a tiered steamer to cook fresh fish and vegetables at the same time.
- Keep fresh fruit and vegetables handy, even at work (keep a fruit bowl on your desk).
- You can add your own fresh vegetables and toppings to pizza bases.
- Always order a starter or side salad when you eat out.
- Make smoothies and fresh juices at home for delicious breakfasts.

Even fresh food can become unhealthy food if it's poorly cooked, so make sure you follow these healthy cooking tips:

- Avoid fried or heavily grilled foods as they can produce free radicals and increase your intake of unhealthy fats. If you must fry, add a small amount of water to cold pressed oil and never let the oil get so hot that it smokes.
- Try grilling or baking instead of frying.
- Avoid aluminium cookware, as this is a heavy toxic metal which can enter food through the cooking process. The same applies to wrapping food in aluminium foil. The best cookware to use is cast iron, enamel, glass or stainless steel.
- To avoid nutrient loss, lightly steam vegetables with a steamer.
- Avoid overcooking food as this can destroy vital nutrients – nutrients you need to fight toxins.
- The toxic effects of microwaving food aren't yet known. Best to avoid.

DETOX SUPERFOODS AND HERBS

Linseeds: a good source of cleansing fibre because they absorb water and expand in the colon, allowing toxins and mucus to be removed. Some people find that ground linseeds, also known as flaxseeds, are an effective remedy for constipation. Flaxseeds also have a lubricating and healing effect on your entire digestive tract.

Grapefruit: has phytochemicals called limonoids that can inhibit tumour formation by promoting the formation of glutathione-S-transferase, a detoxifying enzyme. This enzyme sparks a reaction in the liver that helps to make toxic compounds more water-soluble for excretion from the body. Grapefruit also contains pectin, a form of soluble fibre that forms a gel-like substance in the intestinal tract that can trap fats such as cholesterol.

Lemon juice in water: has a slightly laxative effect and is cleansing to the digestive tract, helping to dissolve mucus and waste. It's high in vitamin C, a powerful antioxidant that helps fight free radical damage and is vital for a healthy immune system. The high potassium content will boost circulation. Potassium also acts as a diuretic and encourages the elimination of nitrogenous waste and chlorides. Squeeze half a lemon into warm water and drink immediately after rising in the morning.

Papaya: wonderful in the aid of digestion. It contains papain, an enzyme that breaks down protein and is very soothing to the stomach and digestive tract. The nutrients in papaya have also been shown to be helpful in preventing colon cancer. In addition, papaya's folate, vitamin C, beta carotene and vitamin E have been associated with a reduced risk of high cholesterol.

Watermelon: thought to be a great detoxifier, diuretic and cleansing agent because it's an excellent source of vitamins C and A, powerful antioxidants that protect against cholesterol and free radical damage. Pink watermelon is also a source of the potent carotenoid antioxidant, lycopene.

Beansprouts: a rich source of detoxifying antioxidant nutrients that protect against free radicals. Sprouts are also a good source of detoxifying fibre and, because of their high concentration of nutrients, are healing and supportive to the digestive system and the body's major detoxifying organ – the liver.

Leafy greens: as well as being a good source of detoxifying and cleansing fibre, leafy greens contain abundant supplies of chlorophyll, one of nature's best cleansers and detoxifiers. Chlorophyll is often taken as a dietary supplement for its ability to combine with gut toxins and remove them from the body. It's also sometimes used as a breath deodorant.

Cabbage: a good source of anti-cancer antioxidants and detoxifying fibre. Research suggests that raw cabbage juice can detoxify the stomach and upper bowels of putrefactive wastes, thereby improving digestive efficiency and facilitating rapid elimination. The antioxidant-responsive element may explain the protective effects of cruciferous vegetables such as broccoli, cabbage and cauliflower on cancer. They are high in substances called indole 3 carbinols which help to prevent oestrogen from being absorbed in the body while at the same time encouraging its elimination.

Soya, lentils, chicken: can naturally reduced the toxic forms of oestrogen in your body and help prevent the risk of diseases such as hypertension.

Fruit and vegetable juices: the cleansers, energizers, builders and regenerators of the human system. A combination of either fresh raw fruit or vegetable juices will supply all the enzymes, vitamins and minerals to aid the body's natural detoxification and increase vitality. (See Dr Sandra Cabot's website www.liverdoctor.com for some practical ideas to boost liver cleansing.)

Nettle tea: a good source of detoxifying chlorophyll. Also has a purifying action on the body when used internally because it helps to remove uric acid from the system – has been used traditionally for the treatment of gout and arthritis. Also has a detoxifying and diuretic effect and helps to clear some of the acids created by junk food diets and rushed lifestyles.

Dandelion tea: contains nutritive salts that can help purify the blood. It's also a diuretic that encourages the flow of urine. The bitter compounds in the leaves and root aid detox by helping to stimulate digestion and acting as mild laxatives. Also increases bile production in the gall bladder and bile-flow from the liver. A great tonic for people with sluggish liver function due to alcohol abuse or a poor diet.

Water: helps the body eliminate waste by making the fibre in food swell. Water is also essential to the digestive process because if we do not drink enough water saliva production slows down and digestion is less efficient. What's more, without water toxins build up in our bloodstream and blood volume decreases, so we have less oxygen and nutrients transported to our cells – all of which can leave us weak, tired and at risk of illness.

Herbal helpers: Alfalfa, burdock, chamomile, dandelion, lemon, red clover, rosehip tea and green tea can all boost liver function and help you gently detox. Sip some throughout the day. Milk thistle is an excellent herb for the liver. Many studies have shown it can increase the number of new liver cells to replace old, damaged ones. Beneficial herbs and spices for the kidneys include goldenrod, cinnamon, cloves, buchu tea and parsley. Numerous herbs support adrenal function, but the most notable are the ginsengs which a qualified practitioner should prescribe (see page 163 for more).

Castor oil: applied externally, can be used to stimulate the liver and draw out toxins from the body. Apply slightly warmed oil to your stomach with a flannel and leave for one hour.

4. PROTECT YOURSELF FROM PESTICIDES

When you pile your plate with vegetables, you get a load of nutrients but you may also get pesticides – chemicals used to protect crops from bugs, rodents and bacteria. And if you use pesticides in your garden or to protect your pets from fleas or to rid your house of rodents, you're exposing yourself as well. They can also be found in some plastics, household products and industrial chemicals. It's estimated that around 359 different pesticides are used in food, on pets or in homes.[10]

Pesticides are potent, extremely toxic chemicals that can interfere with hormonal health. Although we are exposed to pesticides every day, thankfully there are things you can do to protect yourself:

- Rinse, don't soak, fresh fruit and vegetables – it's a more effective way of removing pesticide residue.

- Trim the fat from meats. Some pesticides collect in animal fat.

- Peel fruits and vegetables before using them. Remove and discard the outer leaves of cabbages and other greens. If you buy organic, you need only scrub the skins.

- Eat a wide variety of fruits and vegetables, as specific pesticides are used for specific crops and you'll avoid eating too much of a given pesticide.

- Use home, lawn and garden pesticides sparingly.

- Consider buying organically-grown food. You can find organic produce in most supermarkets these days. If you think organic produce is too expensive, consider buying just one item a week to get you into the habit of looking at it as an investment in your health. Specifically look for organically-grown spinach, peaches, peppers, strawberries, cherries, celery, apples, apricots, green beans, grapes and cucumbers, as according to the US FDA (Food & Drug Administration) the non-organic forms of these foods consistently contain the most pesticides. You could also get mail-order boxes delivered to your door. Make sure the food you buy is really organic by looking for certification labels from well-respected organizations such as the Soil Association (UK) or Earth Source Greens (US). If you eat meat, consider eating only organic. For many years cattle, chickens and even farmed fish have been routinely treated with hormones and antibiotics to keep them healthy and to step up their weight gain. More research is needed, but a growing number of experts believe these hormones may be adversely affecting our hormonal health and increasing the risk of cancer. Organically-produced meat is produced without the routine use of drugs common in intensive livestock farming.

5. PROTECT YOURSELF FROM PLASTICS

We drink from plastic bottles and use plastic food wraps all the time, but a growing number of scientists are getting concerned about the safety of these products, along with tin cans and dental sealants. This is because some substances in certain plastics have been shown to have endocrine-disrupting chemicals (EDCs).

One such chemical is bisphenol-A, used in the manufacture of many food containers, tins, baby bottles and dental sealants. No one knows how this chemical affects humans, but in research on animals it has been shown to have oestrogen-like effects. Other research has raised questions about the safety of cling film made of a type of plastic called polyvinyl chloride (PVC) which contains plasticizers. Some animal studies[11] suggest that PVC may be an endocrine disruptor.

Until we know more about the effects of common plastics on our health, use the simple strategies below to protect yourself:

- Use plastic wraps and cookware made of polyethylene, which doesn't contain plasticizers.
- When you cook or reheat food, don't let plastic wrap touch it.
- Immediately remove cling film wrap from food you buy and transfer to a bag or container. Better yet, ask the person on the deli counter to wrap your food in paper.
- Don't store fatty food in plastic wrap. Xenoestrogens are lipophilic (fat-loving) and will tend to leach into foods with a high fat content.
- If you buy hard cheese wrapped in plastic, use a knife to shave off the surface layer.

- Avoid food that needs to be microwaved in a plastic container. Better still, avoid microwaving altogether.
- Don't wrap your food in cling film; use paper instead.
- Use glass bottles. Cans and plastic bottles of fizzy drink contain six times the amount of aluminium compared to the same beverages in glass bottles. There's always a small amount of residue that dissolves into drinks from the lining of a can or from a plastic bottle. Glass bottles are much better than plastic.

6. DRINK LIGHTLY, OR NOT AT ALL

Alcohol is known to interfere with hormonal balance. If you've got PCOS, drinking too much isn't sensible for the following reasons:

- Alcohol exerts an oestrogen-like action.
- Studies show that women who drink in excess stop ovulating and take longer to get pregnant.
- Alcohol is high in calories and can stop you absorbing zinc, which is crucial for hormonal health.
- Alcoholic drinks are often high in sugar and enter your bloodstream very quickly, which means they can cause rapid fluctuations in blood sugar balance.
- The liver metabolizes alcohol, either converting it to energy or storing it as fat. When too much is consumed this can interfere with the liver's normal functioning and make it less able to clear out excess hormones and toxins.
- Fat builds up in the liver. Since alcohol converts to fat, obesity is common among those who drink to excess.

- Chronic heavy drinking can increase the risk of breast cancer, weaken bones, cause fertility problems and birth defects, and interfere with blood sugar control.

The risks of alcohol are related to the amount you drink. High-risk use would be having more than five drinks daily, moderate risk three to four drinks a day, and low risk one or two drinks daily. If you have PCOS we strongly advise you to cut alcohol out altogether while you're trying to get your symptoms under control. When you're cutting down, follow the healthy eating guidelines described in Part 1 of this book, making sure you eat every two to three hours and drinking lots of water to cleanse your body of toxins.

Once you feel fitter and healthier there's no reason why you shouldn't enjoy the odd glass of wine, spirits or beer. A small amount of alcohol may even be beneficial[12] as it's thought that one or two glasses of red wine a day may decrease the risk of heart disease. This is because red wine contains bioflavonoids, which are cardio-protective. Beer and spirits may have just the same immune-boosting health benefits as wine, but research is always based on moderate to low alcohol intake. No more than one or two drinks a day is ideal.

Drinking alcohol in small amounts regularly could mean you are less likely to become obese than if you do not drink at all, according to a US study published in the December 2005 journal *BMC Public Health*. But the researchers said the results didn't mean teetotallers should turn to the bottle in the battle of the bulge. The study indicated that the odds of overweight and obesity were significantly higher among those who indulged in binge-drinking and/or heavy drinking – four or more drinks per day. In contrast, light to moderate drinking – one or two drinks per day – was associated with lower odds of being overweight or obese.

7. READ LABELS

It's important to pay attention to food labels and get used to spotting hidden ingredients. This is because additives in our food have been linked to a variety of health problems including headaches, asthma, allergies, hyperactivity in kids and even cancer. For women with PCOS, these additives – colourings, preservatives, flavour enhancers, emulsifiers and thickeners – can make the body's own detox system less efficient, add to the toxic load and increase the likelihood of irregular periods, acne, hair loss, weight gain and fatigue.

We are fortunate today that food manufacturers are required to list the ingredients in their products. Despite this, studies show that food labels can still be confusing and misleading for consumers. The following guidelines should make things easier for you.

COLOURINGS

A dangerous class of additives, and one of the easiest to avoid, are the dyes capable of interacting with and damaging your immune system, speeding up ageing and even pushing you in the direction of cancer. Steer clear of foods made with artificial colours. Watch out for labels listing any of the following: 'artificial colour added', the words 'green', 'blue' or 'yellow' followed by a number, 'colour added' with no explanation, tartrazine (E102), quinoline yellow (E104), sunset yellow (E110), beetroot red (E162), caramel (E150) or FD and C red no 3.

Many synthetic food dyes that have initially been deemed safe have turned out to be carcinogenic. Some dyes approved in Europe aren't considered safe in the US and vice versa. You wouldn't add dyes to the food you cook at home, so why eat them in the foods that you buy?

Some foods contain natural colours obtained from plants; these are safe. The most common is annatto, from the reddish seed of a tropical tree. Annatto is often added to cheese to make it more orange, or to butter to make it more yellow. Red pigments, obtained from beets, green from chlorella and carotene from carrots are also OK.

PRESERVATIVES AND FLAVOUR ENHANCERS

The main function of preservatives is to extend a food's shelf-life. Citric acid and ascorbic acid (vitamin C, ascorbates, E300-4) are natural antioxidants added to a number of foods, and they are safe, but synthetic additives such as BHA and BHT (E320-21) may not be. They may promote the carcinogenic changes in cells caused by other substances.

Alum, an aluminium compound, is used in brands of many pickles to increase crispiness and is also found in some antacids and baking powder. Aluminium has no place in human nutrition and you should avoid it.

Nitrates (Nitrites, E249-52) are a type of preservative added to processed meats such as hot dogs, bacon and ham. They can create highly carcinogenic substances called nitrosamines in the body. It's best to avoid any products containing sodium nitrate or other nitrates.

Monosodium glutamate (MSG or 621), a natural product long used in East Asian cooking, is added to many manufactured foods as a flavour enhancer. It's an unnecessary source of additional sodium in the diet and can cause allergic reactions. Omit MSG from recipes, don't buy products containing it, and when eating Chinese request that food be made without it. Other flavour enhancers and preservatives to avoid include monopotassium glutamate (622), sodium osinate (631), benzoic acid and benzoates (E210-9) found in soft drinks, beers and salad creams.

EMULSIFIERS, STABILIZERS, THICKENERS

These are found in sauces, soups, breads, biscuits, cakes, frozen desserts, ice cream, margarine and other spreads, jams, chocolate and milk shakes. They include guar gum (E412), gum arabic (E414), pectins (E440), cellulose (E460), lecithin (E322) and glycerol (E422).

Some chemicals are harmless, for instance ammonium bicarbonate, malic acid, fumaric acid, lactic acid, lecithin, xanathan, guar gums, calcium chloride, monocalcium phosphate and monopotassium phosphate – but how can you tell when there's a long list of chemical names that look unfamiliar to you? A good general rule is simply to avoid products whose chemical ingredients outnumber the familiar ones.

More and more manufacturers are cleaning up their products as people get more concerned about toxins in their food, and you will increasingly see 'no artificial sweeteners' or 'no artificial ingredients' on labels. This is helpful, but still keep an eye out for hidden fats, salts and sugars, and alternative names for ingredients that aren't very good for you when eaten in excess. Sugar names include sucrose, fructose, dextrose, corn syrup, malt syrup and maple syrup. Sodium is just another name for salt, animal fat is saturated fat, and transfatty acid is another name for hydrogenated fat. Mannitol, sorbitol, xylitol, saccharine and aspartame are just alternative names for potentially carcinogenic artificial sweeteners.

If you can't understand a label, or there's barely room for all the chemical ingredients, leave the product on the shelf.

8. DRINK PURE WATER

It's estimated that as many as 60,000 different chemicals now contaminate our water supply. In addition to man-made oestrogens a 2004 report[13] found traces of Prozac and seven other drugs in the UK water supply.

The standard purification techniques used by most water companies remove the bugs from the water but don't remove all the dissolved chemicals. In attempts to clean the water, other chemicals are often added included chlorine and aluminium. Not only may these chemicals be toxic in their own right, but they may react (as in the case of chlorine) with organic waste to form compounds which can increase the risk of cancer of the colon, rectum or bladder.

We've already seen how important it is if you've got PCOS to ensure an adequate intake of fluids. For a detox, water is just as vital because it replenishes, cleanses, rejuvenates and restores your liver, kidneys and adrenals. It's perhaps the most important element of any detoxification plan.

The recognition that much of our tap water is contaminated has seen a boom in bottled water sales. Trouble is, the next bottle of water you drink may be nothing more than tap water that has passed through a filter. There's also little need to drink mineral water. While this type of water does contain minerals, it also contains calcium carbonate which our bodies need but cannot absorb from water. The calcium carbonate can contribute to blockage of the arteries and to indigestion. The best way to up your mineral intake is to eat vegetables grown in mineral-rich soil.

Distilled water isn't much better, as the process can concentrate some compounds and remove essential trace elements. For water to be pure it must be double distilled, and not many companies do this.

The cheapest and easiest way to ensure the water you're drinking is clean and pure is to purify it in your home with water filter systems. Water filter jugs are readily available at supermarkets. Use the filtered water for cooking as well as for hot and cold drinks. Bear in mind that filters can become breeding grounds for bacteria, so regularly replace the filter and clean the jug. A good-quality filter should eliminate or greatly reduce the levels of heavy metals such as lead, cadmium and chlorine and remove any adverse tastes, colours and smells in the water.

Check if your water supply has lead pipes, as lead can leach into the water just by standing in lead pipes overnight. If you have lead pipes, allow your tap to run for a minute first thing in the morning and use water from the cold rather than the hot tap, as lead dissolves more easily in hot water.

If you want to go to the next level you can buy plumbed-in carbon filters for use in your kitchen sink, or you can go for a reverse-osmosis system which is fitted to your mains water system at home. Alternatively, buy water bottled in glass rather than plastic, or simply drink cooled boiled tap water – this at least gets rid of the bacteria and removes the amount of lime scale you're drinking.

9. TOXIC-FREE LIVING

As we've seen, all the chemicals and other toxic substances that we come into contact with in our daily lives can make PCOS symptoms worse and interfere with hormonal health. Since there's a clear link between toxins and hormonal health it makes sense to avoid possible sources of contamination. Toxins can be absorbed through the skin, they are in the air you breathe, in the food that you eat and in the liquid you drink. Fortunately, there are many things you can do to protect yourself.

1. Many perfumes and scented products such as air-fresheners contain worrying chemicals (such as 'artificial musk'). Check toiletries and cosmetics. Be especially wary of the aluminium in deodorants. Use natural cosmetic products and deodorants instead. Treat your pets or your house with natural herbal sprays or garlic – or better still, open a window instead of spraying air-freshener.

2. The same goes for make-up, moisturizers, etc. Explore your local health store or reputable on-line health sites and see what natural alternatives are out there. Tampons, especially super absorbent ones, may dry the vagina – making the transfer of toxins into the vagina easier. Best to use towels instead. If you prefer using a tampon, make sure you change it every four hours. Some studies have found that the only type of tampons that don't produce toxins are the 100 per cent cotton ones.

3. Minimize the amount of polish, bleach, detergents and air-fresheners you use. Try to buy natural products or use tried-and-tested cleaners such as white vinegar and lemon for stain removal, and chemical-free liquid soaps and detergents.

4. See green: At least once a day, try to take a stroll in a park or green place. Trees give out energizing oxygen. It's also a good idea to have plants in your home and workplace. NASA research has shown that the following plants can extract fumes, chemicals and smoke from the air: peace lilies, dwarf banana plants, spider plants, weeping figs, geraniums and chrysanthemums.

5. Refuse and, when possible, replace mercury-containing dental fillings with non-toxic ones. There are also high levels of mercury in tuna fish, so eat it no more than two or three times a week.

6. Devices that emit electromagnetic radiation such as VDUs, mobiles and microwaves should be used with caution and as far away from the bedroom as possible. Buy battery-operated clocks and radios, and unplug electrical goods before you go to bed. Limit your time spent at VDU screens, as some research suggests it can increase the risk of miscarriage. Take regular breaks, around 5 minutes every half hour, and switch the VDU off rather than using the screensaver. An ionizer on top of your desk may help.

7. Many household paints give off dangerous fumes as they dry. Water-based paints are better because they contain fewer 'volatile organic compounds' (VOCs).

8. Toys made from PVC plastic can contain softeners called phthalates which are suspected hormone-disrupters. Ask for PVC-free toys in the shop. (By law, new teething toys should now be free from phthalates.)

9. Plastic baby bottles, beakers and tableware made from polycarbonate can leak potentially risky chemicals when worn or scratched. Replace battered or scratched plastic utensils with new ones.

10. Check chemicals at work. Carbon disulphide, used in several chemical manufacturing processes such as the production of plastics, has been linked to hormonal imbalance. Many pesticides and herbicides are known to contain reproductive toxins. People working in gardens, parks, plant nurseries and farms are at risk. Exposure to heavy metals (traffic fumes), to solvents (dry cleaning, etc.) and to glycol ethers used by electronics-manufacturing firms have been linked to fertility problems.

⇨ DOES USING DEODORANTS RAISE THE RISK OF BREAST CANCER?

The Daily Mail reports that molecular biologist Dr Phillipa Darbre of Reading University has suggested that aluminium compounds used in deodorants may have the same effect on the body's cells as oestrogen, which can help cancers grow. Dr Sarah Rawlings of Breakthrough Breast Cancer says, 'A large number of scientific studies have investigated breast cancer risk factors, however there is no reliable evidence to suggest deodorant or anti-perspirant use – on their own or in combination with shaving – are among them.' Dr Darbre has called for more research to see if a link does exist.[14]

No lifestyle plan for women with PCOS would be complete without taking into account the effect of hormonally-active agents in the environment – whether they are swallowed or inhaled, voluntarily or involuntarily. Taking measures to avoid toxins in the food we eat and the environment we live and work in can help protect us from the added hormonal disturbance and reduce the toxic load.

Does this mean you can never have unfiltered water, eat a non-organic apple or spend hours working on the computer again? Not at all, but remember the 80:20 rule. It applies to detox lifestyle change as well as diet and exercise. If you get it right 80 per cent of the time, you're doing brilliantly. You still have to live in the real world, after all!

Healthy eating, regular exercise and common-sense precautions to avoid overexposure to toxins are, more often than not, sufficient to reduce the risk of toxic overload. Find a balanced, achievable programme, but don't go overboard. Remember you're trying to set up healthy habits to beat symptoms of PCOS – not further stress your body with rapid, extreme and unsustainable changes.

CHAPTER 9
THE BEST NUTRITIONAL AND HERBAL SUPPLEMENTS

A healthy diet, regular exercise and minimizing your exposure to environmental toxins make up the first line of defence against PCOS – but because so many factors are involved in PCOS, taking nutritional supplements can also help.

In theory we should all be getting the nutrients we need from a healthy diet. But, an increasing number of us don't, partly because of poor food choices but also because many high-nutrient foods are just not as nutritious as they used to be due to over-farmed soils, food lying in cold storage for weeks before being put on the supermarket shelves, and so much food being processed. Add to this the extra pressures of modern life on our bodies – in the form of pollution and stress – and it's easy to understand why many of us could benefit from a helping hand in the form of supplements.

Although serious deficiencies of some nutrients are easy to spot (a lack of vitamin C causes gums to bleed, for example), low intakes aren't so easy to detect. Analyses of hair and nail samples aren't always reliable, and getting urine and blood tests isn't always easy. A quicker and easier way to determine if you need to take any supplements is to check out the website of the Health Supplement Information Service (www.hsis.org). Use the nutrition calculator devised by nutritionist Dr Ann Walker to check your intake from each main food group and to give you an idea of which supplements you might benefit from taking.

SUPPLEMENTS DO NOT REPLACE HEALTHY EATING

Everyone should aim to eat as varied and balanced a diet as possible to provide their nutritional needs, avoiding too many fatty and sugary foods. Supplements shouldn't be used as a substitute for a healthy, balanced diet – after all, there's even more to food than vitamins and minerals – fibre, essential fats and protein, for example.

It's also important to get the potential benefits of supplements in proportion. They won't make you feel instantly better, but if you are low in a nutrient, for example iron, they can gradually restore energy levels and concentration in a month or so.

On the other hand, it's possible to overdose on certain supplements: selenium, for instance, has a smallish window between the amount that does you good (up to 200mcg) and the amount that is potentially toxic (more than 900mg). With vitamin A 800mcg a day is OK, whereas taking more than 7,500mcg can cause liver damage. Too much is especially dangerous when pregnant, potentially causing birth defects. And taking too much of one mineral, such as zinc, can lead to poor absorption of others, such as iron and copper. To stop this happening it's vital that you consult a qualified nutritionist to ensure dosages are safe.

Don't let these warnings scare you off, though. Taken at the right time and in the right amounts, supplements can help prevent and control PCOS symptoms in the long term. They can ease the journey through tough times in your life and reduce the risk of the health risks associated with PCOS.

It's best to take most of your supplements as early in the day as possible. You need to take them daily to see and feel improvements, which typically occur after one to three months. Ideally you should have a nutritional therapist make up a prescription for you.

CAUTION

If you're on any kind of medication, have high blood pressure, insulin resistance, are pregnant or hoping to be, consult your doctor before taking supplements of any kind.

YOUR MULTIVITAMIN AND -MINERAL SUPPLEMENT

Finally, after more than 50 years, leading medical journals now recommend that all adults take multivitamins and -minerals. A large body of research has clearly demonstrated that the nutrients found in multivitamins and -minerals reduce your risk of chronic disease, improve quality of life and increase longevity. A multivitamin and -mineral is therefore a good insurance policy if you've got PCOS.

Women with PCOS simply can't afford to be deficient in any of the essential nutrients, so on top of your healthy diet we strongly advise you to consider taking a multivitamin and -mineral supplement containing vitamins A, D, E, C, B_1, B_2, B_3, B_5, B_6, B_{12}, folic acid, vitamins C, D, E, calcium, magnesium, iron, zinc, chromium, selenium and manganese. You may need to take two or more tablets a day to meet your requirements. The bulkiest nutrients are vitamin C, calcium and magnesium, which may need to be taken separately.

KEY NUTRITIONAL AND HERBAL SUPPLEMENTS FOR PCOS

The supplements recommended below have been studied in clinical trials and have suggested positive results in connection with PCOS. Holistic nutritionist Marilyn Glenville recommends:

'A good quality multivitamin and -mineral would form the foundation of your supplement programme to make sure that you're getting a little bit of everything. You then add in other nutrients in slightly higher amounts which are known to be helpful for PCOS.'

Opinion differs among PCOS experts but the most commonly recommended supplements – in addition to a good-quality multivitamin and -mineral – are: the B complex, chromium, and EFAs. To this basic regime other supplements can be added depending on your particular symptoms. We therefore recommend that you consult a licensed healthcare professional regarding the best supplements for you.

Buy your supplements from reputable companies that emphasize quality control and which, if pressed, can supply you with independent analysis of their products. Not all the supplements listed below need to be taken in the long term. For best results you should take them over a period of three months, at the end of which you should be reassessed in order to monitor improvements and changes, and then adjust your supplement programme accordingly.

CHROMIUM

Chromium is an extremely important mineral if you have PCOS. It's an essential nutrient needed for insulin activity in carbohydrate, fat and protein metabolism. Optimal levels may reduce insulin resistance,[1] improve blood sugar control, and reduce the risk of cardiovascular disease, obesity and Type 2 diabetes.[2] Studies[3] show that supplementation with chromium can reduce food cravings, boost efforts at weight loss and help to reduce triglycerides and total cholesterol while improving HDL ('good' cholesterol). Research[4] on women with PCOS and insulin resistance has shown encouraging results with chromium supplementation.

There are a number of different forms of chromium supplements. Chromium polynicotinate appears to have a beneficial effect on glucose metabolism in people with Type 2 diabetes. Chromium picolinate is the generally recommended form of chromium for women with PCOS. Chromium chloride is another common form, but it appears to be less effective than the others. A typical recommended dose of chromium is 200–600mcg per day. However, if you're looking for a therapeutic effect, higher doses might be more effective and work more quickly. Up to 1,000mcg a day is considered safe. Dr Ann Walker recommends 600mcg of chromium GFT for women with PCOS who are insulin resistant.

Brewer's yeast is the richest food source of chromium. It can also be found in liver, mushrooms, wheat germ, oysters, some cheeses, wholewheat bread, beets, fresh fruit and chicken breasts.

VITAMIN B COMPLEX

'The B vitamins are very important in helping to correct the symptoms of PCOS,' says Marilyn Glenville, who treats women with PCOS in her London and Tunbridge Wells clinics.

B vitamins are essential for the liver to convert your 'old' hormones into harmless substances which can then be excreted from the body. Research has also shown that giving women vitamin B_6 increases their fertility. In one study,[5] 12 out of 14 women who had been trying to conceive for seven years conceived after taking vitamin B_6 daily for six months.

Vitamins B_2, B_3, B_5 and B_6 are particularly useful for controlling weight and blood sugar levels. Vitamin B_2 helps to turn fat, sugar and protein into energy. B_3 is a component of the glucose tolerance factor (GTF), which is released every time blood sugar rises, and vitamin B_3 helps to keep the levels in balance. Vitamin B_5 has been shown to help with fat metabolism. B_6 is also important for maintaining hormone balance and, together with B_2 and B_3, is necessary for normal thyroid hormone production. Any deficiencies in these vitamins can affect thyroid function and consequently affect the metabolism.

If you want to take extra B vitamins it's advisable to take a supplement of vitamin B complex rather than separate supplements of each B vitamin. Stress, poor diet, over-exercising, smoking, caffeine, alcohol, exposure to environmental toxins and, in some cases, the Pill can all deplete essential B vitamins. Supplement with one 50-mg vitamin B complex capsule daily.

ANTIOXIDANTS

As mentioned earlier, vitamins A, C, E, beta carotene, zinc, selenium, iron, copper, manganese and the amino acids glutathione and cysteine are known as antioxidants. They are important for skin health and for reducing the risk of insulin resistance, diabetes and cancer. (For more on the remarkable health benefits of antioxidants, see page 90.)

Antioxidants are abundant in fruits, vegetables and sprouted grains, so make sure you get plenty of these foods in your diet. If, however, you exercise a lot and/or are exposed to a lot of stress and chemical pollutants, it might be wise to add an antioxidant complex to your supplement programme. If you're eating a healthy diet and taking a multivitamin and - mineral supplement you may not need to take additional antioxidants unless advised by your doctor or nutritional therapist.

VITAMIN D

Over the past 30 years, numerous studies have established a role for calcium in egg maturation and normal follicular development. PCOS is characterized by hyperandrogenic chronic anovulation (lack of ovulation) due to excess androgens (masculinizing hormones), ovarian theca cell overgrowth, and arrested follicular development. Vitamin D plays a crucial role in calcium absorption and regulation. A study[6] conducted at Columbia University investigated whether vitamin D and calcium dysregulation contribute to the development of follicular arrest in women with PCOS, resulting in reproductive and menstrual dysfunction. They studied 13 women who had chronic anovulation, hyperandrogenism and vitamin D insufficiency. Nine had abnormal pelvic sonograms, with multiple ovarian follicular cysts. All were hirsute, two had hair loss, and five had acanthosis nigricans (patches of darkened skin).

Vitamin D combined with calcium supplementation resulted in normalized menstrual cycles within 2 months for seven of these women. Two became pregnant and the others maintained normal menstrual cycles. These data suggest that abnormalities in calcium balance may be responsible, in part, for the arrested follicular development in women with PCOS, and may contribute to symptoms of PCOS.

Two other recent studies[7] have shown that vitamin D deficiency may be a contributing factor to insulin resistance and diabetes, both of which are problems for women with PCOS. These and other studies suggest that vitamin D plays a role in the secretion, and possibly the action, of insulin.

You can increase your vitamin D levels by taking a multivitamin and - mineral that includes vitamin D, and by exposing your skin to more sunlight. Good food sources include low-fat dairy products, oily fish and fortified milk and cereals. You can also take a vitamin D supplement. Since vitamin D is toxic in high doses, it's wise to get your vitamin D level measured with a blood test, or consult with a licensed naturopathic physician before taking it as a supplement.

CALCIUM

Calcium appears to improve insulin sensitivity. In one study,[8] people taking calcium supplements had reduced insulin levels and improved insulin sensitivity as compared to people who didn't take the supplements.

Recent studies[9] also show that extra calcium helps with weight loss. In animal studies, those given extra dietary calcium or calcium supplements lost more weight than animals with lower calcium intake.

Good sources of calcium include dairy foods, brazil nuts, almonds, sesame seeds, salmon with bones and leafy green vegetables, although calcium from milk and milk products is more easily absorbed and present in greater amounts. If you have trouble consuming enough calcium-rich foods in your daily diet, talk to your doctor or a dietician about using a calcium supplement. The amount of calcium you will need depends on how much calcium you're consuming through food sources.

MAGNESIUM

Magnesium levels have been found to be low in people with diabetes, and there's a strong link between magnesium deficiency and insulin resistance.[10] It's, therefore, an important mineral to include if you have PCOS.

If you want to supplement with magnesium you shouldn't consume more than 600mg a day. Recommended daily intake is in the region of 300mg.

MANGANESE

This mineral helps with the absorption of fats and also works to stabilize blood sugar levels. It also functions in many enzymes including those involved in burning energy. Foods rich in manganese include green leafy vegetables, pecans, pulses and whole grains.

ZINC

Zinc is an important mineral for appetite control; deficiency can cause a loss of taste and smell, creating a need for stronger-tasting foods, including those that are saltier, more sugary and fattier. Zinc is also necessary for the correct action of many hormones, including insulin, so it's extremely important in balancing blood sugar and maintaining a healthy reproductive cycle. It also is excellent for problem skin, and has been suggested for the treatment of depression and eating disorders.

Zinc is one of the key minerals that we need in our daily diets. Unfortunately, because our soil has been depleted by over-farming, there's very little natural zinc found in our food. Furthermore, processing and refining strip out what little might remain. So, no matter how good your diet, you may not be getting anywhere near the levels of zinc that you need.

To boost your intake, eat more whole grains and make sure your multivitamin and -mineral contains zinc. If you don't think you're getting enough you may want to take a daily 15-mg supplement – don't take any more than this, though, as high zinc levels may make you more vulnerable to infections and poor health.

ESSENTIAL FATTY ACIDS/FISH OILS

As we saw in Chapter 6, essential fatty acids (EFAs) are crucial for healthy hormone function and are needed in every cell of your body. They keep your skin soft and smooth, repair damaged skin cells and dissolve fatty deposits that block pores. Studies[11] also suggest that Omega 3 fatty acids can improve insulin sensitivity and reduce insulin resistance.

On top of all this, a diet low in Omega 3 fatty acids is linked to a higher incidence of depression (not surprising when you consider that the human brain is more than 50 per cent fat) and infertility. Given that fatty acids play such a vital role in our health, many researchers believe that a deficiency is a leading cause of cancer and heart disease.

To meet your essential fat requirements, consume 1 or 2 tablespoons of a cold-pressed blend of seed oils providing Omega 3. The other possibility is to supplement with capsules. For Omega 3 this means fish oil capsules or flaxseed or hempseed oil capsules.

As these essential fatty acids are so vital it's advisable, says Dr Marilyn Glenville,

'to supplement them in your diet in the most readily available form. Whatever supplement you choose, read the label on the back of the container and aim for a supplement that gives you at least 150mg of GLA [Omega 6] a day. With EPA [Omega 3] aim for a supplement that will give you at least 2g per day.'

If you're a vegetarian and prefer not to take fish oil, then linseed or hempseed or flaxseed oils contain both Omega 3 and Omega 6.

CO-ENZYME Q10

This is a vitamin-like substance contained in nearly every cell of your body. It's important for energy production and normal carbohydrate metabolism (the way our bodies break down the carbohydrates we eat in order to turn them into energy). One study showed that people on a low-fat diet doubled their weight loss when they supplemented with Co-Q10. Co-Q10 has also proved useful in controlling blood sugar levels.[12]

Co-Q10 is perhaps best known as a heart–healthy supplement. Research has shown it can lower blood pressure, which can reduce the risk of heart attack or stroke. The usual dose is two 60-mg capsules twice a day. Ideally it should be taken under the guidance of a nutritional therapist.

INOSITOL

Recent studies have suggested that women with PCOS may have insulin resistance and hyperinsulinaemia due to a d-chiro inositol deficiency. D-chiro-inositol has been shown to influence the action of insulin.

A study[13] from the Medical College of Virginia found that 1,200mg of d-chiro-inositol daily had multiple beneficial effects in the treatment of 22 overweight women with PCOS. Not only did it improve the action of insulin, but 86 per cent of the women ovulated during treatment compared to only 27 per cent in the placebo group. Serum androgen (male hormone) and ovarian androgen production also decreased in the treatment group. Another study showed similar results in lean PCOS women.

But there's one big problem: D-chiro-inositol isn't commercially available, either as a drug or as a nutritional supplement. Since d-chiro inositol isn't available, what about ordinary inositol, which is readily available?

Studies suggest that this form of inositol may be helpful for PCOS and polycystic ovaries. In one study[14] at the University of Perugia in Italy, 136 women with PCOS took inositol (100mg, twice daily) for 14 weeks. Another group of women took placebo pills. The ovulation frequency was significantly higher in the treated group (23 per cent) compared with the placebo (13 per cent). The time in which the first ovulation occurred was significantly shorter (23.6 days) compared with 41.8 days for the placebo group. The number of patients failing to ovulate was higher in the placebo group. The effect of inositol on follicular maturation was rapid. Also, significant weight loss (and leptin reduction) was recorded in the inositol group, whereas members of the placebo group gained weight.

This all suggests that inositol improves ovarian function in women with irregular cycles and polycystic ovaries.

According to the study above, women appeared to get some benefit from a dose of only 200mg daily, which is a very moderate amount. A considerably higher dose may be appropriate in some situations, but consult with your physician as to how much more you should take. Alternatively you can increase your inositol consumption substantially by consuming more beans. Beans have the added benefit of being a healthy, low-GI food. Another concentrated source of inositol is soy lecithin. Taking a couple of tablespoons of soy lecithin granules daily is a great way to get more inositol.

HERBS

Herbs are extremely useful in the treatment of PCOS. Making changes and adding supplements to your diet will help to control weight and balance blood sugar, while herbs go a step further, targeting any problems involving hormone balance.

Since PCOS is chronic, herbs can help greatly due to the fact that they are much gentler on the body than synthetic drugs. They also have fewer side-effects and many can be used for sustained periods of time.

AGNUS CASTUS (VITEX/CHASTETREE BERRY)

This seems to be the herb most often used by women with PCOS. Vitex has a direct effect on the pituitary gland (involved in regulating hormone production and the menstrual cycle). It's an adaptogen, which means that whether you suffer from a low level of one hormone or an excess of another, you can take Agnus castus and achieve normal levels.

It seems to restore progesterone to a normal level, helpful for those with low levels. Low progesterone levels can cause miscarriage, so vitex can help to prevent this. It's also used for irregular menstruation, amenorrhoea and PMS. Side-effects include digestive upsets and a mild rash with itching.

Available from health food stores, herbalists and nutritional therapists, it should be taken for a period of several months to determine efficacy. A typical recommended dose of Vitex organic tincture is 1 teaspoon, 3 times a day for 3 or 4 months. The herb can be taken daily for up to 18 continuous months, unless pregnancy occurs.

If you decide to take Vitex, always check with your doctor first. If depression is one of your symptoms you should probably avoid it, as some research suggests that PMS depression may be related to excess progesterone, and Agnus castus can raise progesterone levels. [15–20]

BLACK COHOSH

Black Cohosh is a uterine tonic herb and exhibits an oestrogenic effect. It's widely used in menopausal formulas but is valuable for treating amenorrhoea, irregular menstruation and symptoms of the menopause and PMS. [21] It's also thought to lower blood pressure and cholesterol levels and improve thyroid function.

DONG QUAI (ANGELICA)

No studies on women with PCOS have been done, but dong quai is similar to vitex, and can be used for long periods of time because it's a tonic herb. It nourishes the liver and endocrine system and may be useful for irregular menstruation, PMS, period pain and menopausal symptoms. It's widely used among Chinese women because of its reputation as a libido and energy booster, and has been dubbed 'the female ginseng'.

CINNAMON

Cinnamon may be very useful for treating the insulin resistance that frequently accompanies PCOS. Several new studies[22] indicate that this delicious spice can lower blood glucose levels.

A recent press release from the University of California, Santa Barbara, Iowa State University and the US Department of Agriculture stated that 'Cinnamon may be more than a spice – it may have a medical application in preventing and combating diabetes. Cinnamon may help by playing the role of an insulin substitute in Type 2 diabetes.'

Study dosages ranged from a quarter teaspoon to 1 teaspoon per day for people with Type 2 diabetes, but more research is needed. The active chemical is MHCP or methylhydroxychalcone polymer. This chemical is found in all types of cinnamon sold as a spice in the US (*Cinnamomum cassia*). However, true cinnamon is *Cinnamomum zeylanicum*, or *Cinnamomum verum*.

MHCP has been shown to lower blood glucose levels, triglycerides and LDL ('bad') cholesterol. It's also known as an antioxidant.

The potential benefits of cinnamon are enormous when you consider how inexpensive it is. Many people who cannot afford expensive diabetes drugs may one day be treated with cinnamon. Try adding a teaspoon a day to cereal, hot porridge with raisins, baked apples or even mashed banana on wholegrain toast.

ECHINACEA

One of the most widely researched of all herbs, Echinacea has broad antibiotic properties,[23] much like penicillin, and is useful for treating acne. You can find alcohol-free tinctures in most health food shops.

EVENING PRIMROSE

Some women with PCOS use evening primrose for PMS, fibrocystic breast disease, bloating, mood swings and to improve skin quality. It's rich in GLA and linolenic acid – essential fatty acids which the body requires to regulate hormones – and may help irregular cycles.

Evening primrose oil is prescribed in the UK under the brand name Efamest. The dose recommended by doctors is around 1,000mg per day. Do bear in mind that not all PCOS experts recommend Evening primrose. According to medical herbalist and nutrition scientist Dr Ann Walker, who treats many women with PCOS: 'Breast pain is perhaps the only indication for evening primrose oil for women with PCOS, although it's also well known for improving skin … Far better to aim for 2 g a day of Omega 3 from fish oil or linseed.'

FENUGREEK

Fenugreek appears to lower blood sugar levels by interfering with the digestion and absorption of sugars and improving the body's use of sugar once it's absorbed. Studies[24] report that fenugreek improves glucose tolerance in people with Type 2 diabetes. A dose of 25 to 50mg of fenugreek seed powder twice daily with meals is typically recommended.

GARCINIA CAMBOGIA

Garcinia cambogia is a small tropical fruit called the 'Malabar tamarind'. It comes from central Asia, where the rind is used in Thai and Indian cooking. The garcinia contains HCA (hydroxy-citric acid) which enables carbohydrates to be turned into usable energy instead of being deposited as fat. The HCA in this fruit seems to curb appetite, reduce sugar cravings and insulin resistance, and inhibit the formation of fat and cholesterol.

GYMNEMA SYLVESTRE

Native to India, this herb comes to us from the Ayurvedic healing tradition (see page 174). It seems to improve insulin sensitivity[25] and, like fenugreek, can also interfere with sugar absorption. In contrast to fenugreek, the doses used for gymnema are only 400–500mg daily.

Other Ayurvedic herbs believed to boost insulin production include turmeric, tulsi, and bitter melon.

MILK THISTLE (SILYBUM MARIANUM)

This is one of the key herbs for the liver (for more on looking after this essential detox organ, see page 130),[26] and is therefore essential for the treatment of PCOS. It helps to protect your liver cells against damage and to promote the healing of damaged cells, so improving the general functioning of the liver and all its detoxifying properties.

Research[27] in 2005 by a group of Southern California researchers suggests that women with PCOS are at increased risk of developing non-alcoholic fatty liver disease (NAFLD), making milk thistle an important herb in the fight against this illness.

Many natural therapists recommend up to three 500-mg tablets of capsules daily for women with PCOS, to help them gently detox. This potent liver-protector is also helpful for symptoms of PMS, acne, stress and fatigue and is an important preventative herb if you smoke, drink alcohol or live in a polluted area.

⇨ 'NATURAL' PROGESTERONE

Although applied topically to the skin rather than taken internally, natural progesterone creams – natural not because they come from a plant but because they're nature-identical chemical formula – allow you to absorb a chemically-produced progesterone that is identical to the hormone produced in your body (rather than being a slightly different chemical mix, known as progestogen). Progesterone plays a major role in regulating menstruation. Progesterone can decrease the risk of endometrial cancer – particularly relevant for women with PCOS. Many women with PCOS have had success using progesterone cream to stimulate periods. A typical dose is a quarter to half teaspoon of natural progesterone cream applied twice daily.

Unfortunately, there are some potential downsides to progesterone creams as well. Since such creams are typically made by independent compounding pharmacies, the creams aren't standardized. Thus, there can be no guarantee of the amount of progesterone present in each batch of cream. As a result, it's particularly important to find a pharmacy of exceptional quality. Also, as with most creams, the amount of hormone delivered throughout the body is unpredictable. This is because the hormone has to be absorbed through your skin and into your blood. The amount that gets into circulation for distribution to other parts of your body depends on the thickness and temperature of your skin, and can vary markedly from individual to individual, making it hard to predict the effect it will have. Therefore, when using the cream it's imperative to get specific instructions from your doctor or pharmacist and then follow those directions consistently.

While problems may or may not arise from using hormone medications, a healthy diet is guaranteed to normalize your hormones without any side-effects at all.

RHODIOLA ROSEA

This powerful Russian nutrient is also an adaptogenic herb thought to help women with PCOS to cope with stress. Research[28] has shown that it can boost libido, help to raise energy levels, boost immunity and aid the detoxification of hormones before they are eliminated from the body. It's also thought to have revitalizing properties and to help stabilize mood swings. Most health food shops now stock this stress-busting adaptogen.

SARSAPARILLA

Thought to help reduce acne and redress hormonal imbalance, Sarsaparilla contains a steroid-like substance that acts in a similar way to progesterone in the body. It's believed to stimulate the reproductive organs and have a tonic-like effect on the sex organs.

ST JOHN'S WORT

Probably the most powerful natural antidepressant. For more information, see Chapter 16, 'Coping with Depression and Low Moods'.

SAIREI-TO

This Chinese herbal medicine may be a useful treatment for women with PCOS and irregular periods, according to research[29] from Japan.

SAW PALMETTO (SERENOA REPENS)

Traditionally used for male prostate problems. Numerous studies[30] have confirmed that saw palmetto is effective in slowing down the conversion of testosterone. As it works as an anti-androgen, it can be very helpful for women with PCOS.

Typically, saw palmetto is suggested to women with PCOS who have excess hair growth, or have been told they have high levels of androgens.

Doses will vary from woman to woman depending on the severity of symptoms, so it's always best to consult with a qualified medical herbalist rather than self-prescribing.

SIBERIAN GINSENG

Known as an adaptogenic herb (adapting itself to your individual needs), Siberian ginseng is believed to help the body adapt to stress, including the metabolic stress of fluctuating blood glucose levels. Currently research is focusing on ginseng as a possible replacement for insulin in treating diabetes. Canadian scientists have found that ginseng taken before or after eating can reduce blood sugar levels significantly.

Ginseng also aids in moving fluids and nutrients around the body. Generally it's best to take ginseng first thing in the morning, as some women have trouble sleeping if they take it later in the day. According to research from Germany, ginseng can on rare occasions raise blood pressure – so it's a good idea to have your blood pressure monitored first as women with PCOS have an increased risk of blood pressure problems. A typical daily dose is 100 to 200mg of a standardized ginseng product.

SPAGYRIC HERBAL REMEDIES

Developed for women with PCOS who are hoping to conceive and cannot use saw palmetto to help redress their underlying hormone imbalances, spagyric formulations ('spagyric' refers to healing forces in nature, such as plants and minerals, applied as remedies and displaying therapeutic effects) include the root of an African plant called *Okoubaka aubrevillei*. They are thought to help clear toxins from the body and can reduce the unexplained weight gain common among women with PCOS. This family of herbs also includes elder, which works specifically to correct hereditary disorders and reduce cysts. The most important, however, is wild yam,[31] which acts as a hormone regulator to restore a normal menstrual cycle and fertility.

UNKEI-TO

This Japanese herbal mixture[32] is a blend of 12 herbs including ginseng, evoida fruit and ginger stem, which can help encourage ovulation in women with PCOS and improve menstrual regularity, thus reducing the risk of endometrial cancer.

The supplements listed here are by no means the only ones recommended for PCOS symptoms, they are simply the ones most often recommended by experts or used by women with PCOS. As you'll see in the next chapter, a number of other supplements can be helpful depending on your symptoms.

A Word of Caution

Whatever herbs or supplements you're considering, be sure to tell your doctor, especially if you're on any kind of medication. There can sometimes be serious drug–herb-supplement interactions. Even if you aren't on medication, it's a good idea to check with your doctor, nutritionist or medical herbalist before taking any herbs or supplements.

CHAPTER 10
HOW NATURAL THERAPIES CAN HELP YOU

Recent studies[1] have confirmed the age-old notion that the mind and body are closely linked. For complementary and alternative treatments, the mind–body connection that scientists are finally confirming often forms the basis of diagnosis and treatment.

COMPLEMENTARY THERAPIES

You may think of complementary therapies as 'alternative' therapies, but this term is misleading as they aren't intended to be used *in place of* conventional medicine. As with improving your diet and environment, complementary therapies should be used *in conjunction with* the treatment and advice given by your doctor. Perhaps one of the best things about complementary therapies is that the therapist is able to spend time with the patient and can usually give you more support than overstretched doctors can.

Complementary therapies are great for women with PCOS because they are non-invasive and can be used in addition to long-term medication. They are also often enjoyable and, in most cases, allow you to relax. In addition, they place the emphasis on preventative medicine, i.e. preventing illness before it happens, which is beneficial for women with PCOS and their increased risk of heart disease, diabetes and infertility. Last but by no means least, natural therapies are suitable for women with PCOS because they treat mind, body and spirit, not just your symptoms, so can help you feel mentally and emotionally energised as well as physically improved.

WHERE TO BEGIN?

The power of natural remedies to improve your health and quality of life relies on identifying which remedy works best for you and your symptoms. With so many alternative therapies available it can sometimes be hard to know where to start. Use the information in this chapter to begin your exploration of natural options. Consult your doctor about alternative therapies. Find a PCOS support group and ask lots of questions. We've always found that the experiences of other women with PCOS can be extremely helpful, but do bear in mind that PCOS affects each one of us differently and what works for one woman may not work for another.

Whatever therapy you decide upon, if you decide upon one, be sure to monitor its effectiveness. Keep a record and pay close attention to your weight, menstrual cycle and other symptoms. Decide in advance how long you want to try a particular therapy before changing your approach.

We have both found natural therapies (TCM, reflexology, herbalism and aromatherapy) extremely beneficial for treating our symptoms, in addition to healthy eating, regular exercise and trying to minimize exposure to environmental toxins. And even if you only decide to dip your toe in now and again with an aromatherapy bath or a soothing, warming herbal tea at the end of the day, it can all help give life with PCOS a positive boost.

ACUPUNCTURE

Acupuncture is a 3,000-year-old traditional form of Eastern healing that involves very fine, sterile, disposable stainless steel needles inserted at selected acupuncture points. These points are located along energy channels (meridians) believed to correspond to specific internal organs.

The practice of acupuncture is based on the understanding that a vital energy called *chi* (or *qi*) flows along these meridians throughout the body. It is thought that if *chi* is blocked or obstructed in its flow, pain or dysfunction may occur. Needles are inserted to increase, decrease or unlock the flow of *chi* energy so that the balance of yin and yang can be restored.

Yin, the female energy force, is calm and passive; it also represents dark, swelling and moisture. Yang, the male force, is stimulating and aggressive; it represents heat, light and dryness. It's thought that an imbalance between these two forces triggers illness. So, for example, if you feel the cold and suffer a lot from fluid retention and fatigue, you would be considered to have an excess of yin. If you get headaches a lot and are quick to lose your temper, you would have an excess of yang.

There are hundreds of acupuncture points, and each point has a predictable therapeutic effect. Problems can be addressed by needling points close to and distant from the problem being treated, because the meridians run throughout the body. For example, a headache may be treated by placing needles in the head, hands and/or feet.

Emotional, physical and environmental forces are all thought to upset the balance of *chi*, and acupuncture is often used to treat stress, digestive disorders, insomnia, addiction, asthma and allergies. It's also thought to be able to kick-start menstrual periods and to help regulate the menstrual cycle in women with PCOS and fertility problems.

DOES ACUPUNCTURE WORK?

The World Health Organization has developed a list of conditions that have proven to be treatable by Oriental medicine and acupuncture. The list contains physical injuries and numerous disorders including ear, nose, eye, throat, gastrointestinal, gynaecological, musculoskeletal, neurological, psychiatric, skin, cardiovascular and respiratory disorders. Western doctors[2] theorize that acupuncture somehow releases the body's natural pain-killers, called endorphins, and a growing number recommend it to alleviate stress. There's also a growing body of evidence that supports its effectiveness for women with PCOS and irregular periods.

A study[3] at Goteborg University in Sweden showed that acupuncture may help some women with PCOS to ovulate. In this study, electro-acupuncture was used instead of traditional acupuncture. Electro-acupuncture, the application of a pulsating electrical current to acupuncture needles as a means of stimulating the acupuncture points, was developed in China as an extension of hand manipulation of the acupuncture needles.

Twenty-four women with PCOS and infrequent or absent periods were included in this study. After 10–14 treatments for two to three months, nine women (38 per cent) experienced regular ovulation. However, the electro-acupuncture wasn't effective in the more severe cases (women who were obese, had the highest waist-to-hip ratio, and highest testosterone and insulin levels). Researchers concluded from the study that, for women with mild PCOS, acupuncture may help induce ovulation.

▷ A VISIT TO AN ACUPUNCTURIST

A qualified acupuncturist will first of all want to talk to you about your lifestyle, sleeping and eating patterns, fears and reactions to stress, as well as any health concerns. Your pulse will be taken and then the treatment will be carried out.

Upon insertion of an acupuncture needle people may experience varying sensations, ranging from no pain at all to a slight pinch, a feeling of heaviness, warmth and achiness or possibly tingling and an electric sensation. The needles are left inserted for 20–45 minutes, and people often become deeply relaxed, and sometimes even fall asleep. After the needles are removed you may feel energized, sleepy or lighter. You may notice immediate improvement of your symptoms.

Women with PCOS can expect to have needles placed in points along their arms, legs and abdomen. The acupuncturist will normally work on the liver and spleen *chi* to treat irregular periods.

The number of acupuncture treatments depends on the duration, severity and nature of your symptoms. If no benefits are noticed after four to six sessions, however, it's probably best to discontinue treatment.

AROMATHERAPY

Plant essences have been used for centuries for the treatment of disease. Aromatherapists work to restore hormonal balance in women with PCOS and to aid relaxation and release emotional stress. Concentrated aromatic oils – known as essential oils – are extracted from plants and are inhaled, rubbed directly onto the skin or used in massage or bathing oils.

There are few clinical trials proving the efficacy of aromatherapy, but those who have used this treatment have no doubt that it works. The oils stimulate the sense of smell, which then affects the part of the brain known as the limbic system. This is connected to mood control, strong emotions, and instinctive behaviour.

Aromatherapy is now a popular treatment in hospitals, hospices, and homes for the elderly. It can bring about feelings of great peace and pleasure, and is an excellent antidote to many of the conditions linked with older age, including depression, insomnia, anxiety and arthritis.

Essential oils can be used in several ways:

Inhalation – place 1 to 5 drops on a handkerchief, in a vaporizer or diffuser, or on a light-bulb ring and inhale the aroma.

Baths – add 4 to 6 drops (no more than 20) of essential oil to 1 teaspoon (5 ml) of carrier oil (such as sweet almond, wheatgerm, olive, apricot kernel, avocado or other plant or vegetable oil), add to bathwater and stir vigorously.

Massage – add 1 to 5 drops of essential oil to 1 teaspoon (5ml) of carrier oil and massage into the affected area. Warming the oil increases absorption.

Compresses – add 3 to 5 drops of essential oil to 300 ml of hot/warm water. Soak a clean flannel or soft cloth in the water, wring out and apply to

affected part of the body (cold for bruises, sprains, headaches; warm for
abscesses, boils, period pains, cystitis). Repeat two to three times a day
until the condition improves.

Steam treatments — add 1 to 2 drops of essential oil to a medium-sized bowl of
freshly boiled water. Cover head with cloth, lean over the water and
inhale the steam, taking care to keep the bowl steady and to not get too
close to the water to prevent scalding.

Gargles and mouthwashes — add 1 to 3 drops to a tumbler of water and stir
vigorously before gargling or rinsing round the mouth. Spit out — don't
swallow.

Some oils shouldn't be used if you're epileptic, have asthma or high blood
pressure, or are pregnant or hoping to be. We've indicated where you need
to proceed with caution. The following list is for general guidance only;
always check with a qualified practitioner before using an aromatherapy oil.

Essential Oil	Use as	To Treat
Bergamot	massage oil, bath oil or in a burner	anxiety, depression, eczema, dermatitis, to lift spirits
Cedar	massage oil, inhalant or bath oil	nervous tension and anxiety
Camomile	massage oil, inhalant or bath oil	anger, irritability, period pains, heavy periods, menopausal problems, insomnia, indigestion
Jasmine	massage oil, bath oil, perfume or in a burner	depression, lack of confidence, impotence, loss of libido, emotional coldness

Essential Oil	Use as	To Treat
Lavender	massage oil, bath oil, inhalant, in a burner or as perfume	anxiety, insomnia, eczema, dermatitis
Rose	massage oil, bath oil or perfume	anxiety, emotional trauma, irregular menstruation, impatience, confusion
Rosewood	massage oil, bath oil or perfume	anxiety, insomnia, mood swings, menstrual pain or irregularity
Sandalwood	bath oil or perfume	stress and irritability
Ylang ylang	massage oil, bath oil, perfume or in a burner	depression, anger, impotence, loss of libido, hypertension, palpitations

Aromatherapist Katherine Ginsberg, co-founder of The Birth Connection (www.birthconnection.co.uk), a group of London-based complementary therapists specializing in menstrual and fertility problems, explains that

'essential oils are often balancing in their effects, helping the body to return to a state of imbalance which has led to illness to one of balance and health. This is one of the reasons why aromatherapy lends itself so well to the treatment of PCOS – which is all about the under- or over-production of various hormones, and the work I do with my clients is often about bringing the body and mind back into balance. Once this has been achieved, the symptoms of PCOS will often improve. Moreover, when essential oils are breathed in they go directly to the brain, the control centre of the hormonal system.'

Joanna Levett, an aromatherapist with PCOS who treats women with PCOS, suggests this aromatherapy massage blend to balance hormones:

In 20 ml carrier oil:

- 2 drops fragrant Jasmine
- 3 drops balancing Geranium
- 3 drops Clary sage (a sedative oil good for absent periods or period pains)

⇨ A VISIT TO AN AROMATHERAPIST

Like acupuncture, aromatherapy is a holistic treatment (it looks at the person as a whole, not just his or her symptoms), and you should expect questions about your lifestyle at a consultation. Depending on your answers an essential oil or two or three (or more) will be recommended.

The massage itself can release powerful emotions and tensions, so don't be surprised to find yourself wiped out but very relaxed after a treatment. You may have a mild adverse reaction, say a headache, but this will pass in a day or two.

If you have hypersensitive skin, you will need to be careful about which oils you use. You also need to learn how to dilute oils in a carrier base – neat oils should never come into contact with the skin.

Warning: If you have high blood pressure, epilepsy, skin disorders, are pregnant or hoping to be, or if you're taking certain homoeopathic medicines, you will need to avoid some oils. Always consult a qualified aromatherapist. Never apply oil to areas of the skin that have been damaged, or to open wounds. Some oils can be phototoxic, so check that it's safe to be out in the sun after a treatment.

If you would prefer not to consult a qualified aromatherapist, your local health food store or chemist may be able to provide you with essential oils that are suitable for your needs. You might also like to buy or borrow an aromatherapy book from your local bookstore or library, or search the Internet for more information.

AUTOGENIC THERAPY

Autogenic therapy has been used with success to treat physical and emotional symptoms of stress, and illnesses exacerbated by stress.[4] It draws on the insights of meditation and is particularly useful for mild anxiety states. The techniques have been found to lower blood pressure and improve emotional balance, both of which are particularly helpful for women with PCOS.

A typical session involves a series of exercises designed to focus your mind on feelings of heaviness and warmth in the limbs, a calm heartbeat, easy natural breathing, and abdominal warmth and cooling of the forehead. You repeat the exercises three times a day after meals for about 10 minutes.

To contact an autogenic training practitioner, see Resources chapter, page 385.

AYURVEDA

Ayu means life and *Veda* means knowledge, therefore *Ayurveda* means the science of life. Ayurveda is the traditional Indian health system which is more than 5,000 years old.

HOW DOES THE AYURVEDIC SYSTEM WORK?

Ayurveda holds that the body has certain rhythms, similar to those found in nature. When these rhythms are balanced the body is healthy; when they are imbalanced the body becomes sick. This system is governed by *Dosha*, the biological force, humour or constitution. There are three different types of Dosha, and all need to be present to create balance in the body. If one is too low or too high, this produces imbalance. This imbalance is called *Vikriti*, while the balance is called *Prakriti*.

The three types of Dosha are:

1. *Vata* – the air type, which governs all movements in the body and mind – for example, breathing, heart beat, elimination, pulsation, blood circulation, and thinking. When the air element is too high, all of the things listed above will increase and the person will become sick or imbalanced.
2. *Pitta* – the fire/heat type. This is responsible for metabolism and digestion. Without adequate heat, your food cannot be properly digested and will become toxic in your system. Pitta is also responsible for keeping the body warm.
3. *Kapha* – the water type. It's responsible for lubrication in the body (joints, skin, mouth) and provides stability.

Everybody is composed of a mixture of all three doshas, though one will be dominant. To get an accurate assessment of your dosha you should consult an Ayurvedic practitioner.

Treatment plans would vary according to individual symptoms, but for women with PCOS might include the following herbal and lifestyle recommendations:

- Castor oil packs – Four applications a week for 1 hour for up to six months to clear obstruction in the pelvis
- Guggul Plus formula – contains Indian myrrh, fennel, fenugreek, trikatu, triphala and rjuna, to normalize metabolism and boost weight loss
- Organic Triphala – helps cleanse the bowel and assist detoxification
- Shatavari – brings balance and strength to the menstrual system
- EFAs – to help restore hormonal balance
- Karela/Bitter melon *(Momordica charantia)* – reduces blood sugar without increasing insulin; appears to enhance tissue sensitivity to insulin
- Fenugreek *(Trigonella foenicum-graecum)* – reduces blood sugar without increasing insulin
- Gurmar *(Gymnema sylvestre)* – helps to reduce blood sugar levels
- Nervines – to help with the stress of amenorrhoea (lack of periods) and infertility. Organic Ashwagandha may be useful here.
- Fibre – reduces fasting blood glucose without increasing insulin
- Chromium picolinate (200–400mcg/day) – black pepper is high in chromium and can assist in balancing blood sugar levels
- Psyllium – reduces post-meal glucose and insulin levels
- Exercise – to enhance tissue sensitivity to insulin (80 per cent of the body's sugar uptake occurs in the muscles)

▷ VISITING AN AYURVEDIC PRACTITIONER

In the initial consultation, which is for a minimum of an hour, a pulse diagnosis would be done. This is to assess the amplitude, rhythm, volume, temperature, movement and strength of your pulse. Your eyes are also checked for their colour, shape, movement and shine. Tongue diagnosis is done to check the colour, coating, thickness, shape and surface. The breathing is observed to watch its rhythm; for example slow, rapid, deep, shallow, long or short. The breath is checked to see its temperature, moisture and how far it can be felt from the nose. The skin surface is also touched to assess whether it's soft, dry, rough, smooth, cold, warm, clammy, moist or oily. Your aura is read and your face diagnosed by looking at its shape. Questions about lifestyle and diet would be asked. You will be asked about your menstrual cycle and any previous pregnancies. Through checking all of these things and asking questions, a proper assessment can be made and the relevant medicine and lifestyle/diet advice can be given.

HERBAL MEDICINE

Herbal remedies have been used for centuries to treat illnesses and boost health and well-being. In fact, 30 per cent of modern conventional medicines are made from plant-derived substances. However, because conventional medicines often have unpleasant and unwanted side-effects, some women with PCOS prefer to use herbal alternatives instead. They rate among the most popular natural therapies for women with PCOS.

Although herbal remedies are natural it's important that they are used with caution because they can interact with certain medications. It's important to inform your doctor if you want to take any herbal remedies, and many doctors believe herbal remedies should only be taken on the advice of a trained herbalist.

A medical herbalist will take a detailed look at your diet and lifestyle. He or she will then write a prescription according to your individual needs. Tablets made from compressed herbal extracts are often prescribed, but sometimes you may be given a bag of carefully weighed and ground dried roots, flowers, bark and so on, with instructions on how to use them, for example in tea.

A number of herbs are considered helpful for women with PCOS and you can find a list of them in Chapter 9 (page 156).

HOMOEOPATHY

Homoeopaths believe that a person's personality and lifestyle determine the disorders he or she may be susceptible to and the symptoms that are likely to encounter.

Homoeopathic remedies are derived from plant, mineral and animal substances which are soaked in alcohol to extract what are known as 'live' ingredients. This initial solution is then diluted many times, shaken to add energy at each dilution. Low dilution remedies are used for severe symptoms, while high dilution remedies are used for milder solutions. After a consultation a homoeopath will offer you a remedy suited to your symptoms, temperament and personality.

HOMOEOPATHIC REMEDIES FOR PCOS

It's because of this variation between one individual to another that there are no specific homoeopathic remedies for the treatment of PCOS. However, the single factor that remains constant is that all cases of PCOS require *constitutional* homoeopathic treatment.

Constitutional treatment requires a remedy that has been selected to treat the individual as a whole. This includes not just PCOS symptoms but everything about you – your personality, food likes and dislikes, weather/seasonal likes and dislikes, sleep patterns and body temperature, to name but a few. Once selected, the appropriate remedy is often prescribed in a very short dosage regime, to act as a short sharp shock to the body's energy system in order to get it vibrating at the right frequency. Follow-ups, to assess the result of the treatment, are usually carried out four to five weeks later.

Constitutional remedies often prescribed for PCOS include Pulsatilla, Nat. mur., Lycopodium, Sepia and Lachesis.

Looking at the diet and nutritional state of the patient is also very important, and some homoeopaths refer PCOS patients to a clinical nutritionist for a full assessment. Although homoeopathic remedies are safe and non-addictive, at first you may find that you feel worse. This is known as a 'healing crisis' and is short lived – and often an indication that the remedy is working.

Some women with PCOS have reported that their periods normalized within six months of taking prescribed homoeopathic remedies, but this information comes from uncontrolled clinical trials. Although studies[5] have reported the positive health benefits of homoeopathy for a range of chronic conditions, the benefits for women with PCOS have yet to be scientifically validated.

NUTRITIONAL THERAPY

Nutrition therapy is the science of proper diet, lifestyle strategies and therapeutic nutrients to correct nutritional insufficiencies, promote optimal health and prevent, manage or correct medical problems. Nutritional therapists often work along side orthodox doctors to boost health and prevent or reverse problems such as high cholesterol, hypertension or high blood pressure, and non-insulin dependent diabetes.

Research has shown that many medical conditions and illnesses, including PCOS, can be managed, improved and even corrected by changes to the diet. Nutritional therapy is a way of using food and supplements to encourage the body's natural healing. It does this by:

- detoxifying the body
- correcting vitamin and mineral deficiencies
- restoring healthy digestion
- developing a positive attitude.

In order to achieve these goals, a nutritional therapist will ask a lot of questions about all aspects of your health and well-being including your medical history, dietary history, family history, menstrual problems, digestion, energy levels and exercise. This helps the therapist discover if you have any problems such as food allergies, nutritional deficiencies, toxic overload or general nutritional problems. Besides asking questions the therapist might suggest doing tests such as a hair mineral analysis, hormone tests or food intolerance tests. The therapist will then suggest foods you should eat and foods to be avoided. They may also recommend a specific type of diet. Supplements and lifestyle changes may be suggested to encourage your body to heal itself.

Nutritional therapies can help to regulate blood sugar and insulin levels, reduce circulating androgens, improve ovarian function, improve fertility, reduce the risk of heart disease and support liver detoxification. As we've seen throughout this book, changing your diet is a powerful and potent way to manage PCOS and the foundation stone of all other treatments.

Depending on your specific presentation of PCOS, a natural therapist will consider a variety of nutritional therapies and supplements and you'll find most of them in Chapter 6 (see page 64) and Chapter 9 (see page 144).

REFLEXOLOGY

Reflexology is an ancient Eastern therapy that is now extremely popular in the West. Experts in this type of manipulative therapy claim that all the organs of the body are reflected in the feet. So in a similar way to accupuncture, reflexology aims to stimulate organs through specific points on the feet.

Experts claim that reflexology aids in the removal of waste products and blockages within the energy channels, improving circulation and glandular function. By applying pressure in the form of a specialized foot massage, a practitioner can determine which energy pathways are blocked.

Reflexology is a popular choice for women with PCOS, not just as a stress-buster but also because it's wonderfully relaxing and thought to be able to help regularize periods and improve circulation. Many therapists prefer to take a full case history before starting treatment. Each session lasts about forty minutes and you will be treated sitting or lying down.

UK-based reflexologist Jacqui Garnier, who has PCOS herself and uses reflexology to help other women, says:

'Reflexology is one of the most effective ways of rebalancing the entire endocrine system. It is particularly successful when used in combination with a healthy diet and lifestyle. As a balancing treatment it has been shown to have success rates as high as 88 per cent in infertility, it can regulate cycles, encourage ovulation and reduce the stress so often associated with coping with the symptoms of PCOS.'

TRADITIONAL CHINESE MEDICINE

Traditional Chinese Medicine (TCM) addresses imbalances in the body with the aim of preventing disease in the future – it is this that makes it particularly helpful for women with PCOS. It can help re-establish the proper functioning of the body and hormones with methods that are gentler and subtler than those of contemporary medicine. It has a whole range of therapeutic techniques at its disposal, including herbs, acupuncture and diet. PCOS expert and acupuncturist Jo George, who runs the Life Medicine Acupuncture and Herb Clinic in London, says:

> 'Treatment with a Chinese practitioner can provide women with PCOS with enough strength to make the necessary changes to our lifestyle. All of us can benefit from simple adjustments, and for many this can mean increased vitality, greater well-being, better hormonal balance and feeling more contented with our lives.'

TCM reports fantastic results with hormonal disturbances, including PCOS, and practitioner Zita West, a former NHS midwife and now a fertility expert who specializes in holistic health for women, says she has helped many PCOS sufferers with TCM and a combination of acupuncture and rebalancing herbal and vitamin supplements.

CHAPTER 11
HOW TO MANAGE YOUR WEIGHT

Weight control for women with PCOS can be a major turning-point for keeping other symptoms at bay.[1] PCOS expert Stephen Frank, Professor of Reproductive Endocrinology at Imperial College, London, says: 'Weight reduction remains the best way for women with PCOS to manage their symptoms and reduce the risk of poor health in the long term.'

If you're already following our advice on healthy eating, exercise and taking care not to overload your body with toxins, the chances are you'll be balancing your hormones, and losing weight as a result.

Having said all that, there's no denying that many women with PCOS do struggle with their weight. Have you ever been told by a friend, loved one or your doctor that you could do with losing weight? And did you feel like yelling, 'You don't say!' Perhaps you want to say, 'You won't believe me but I don't eat that much now. How can I eat even less?' This is one of the most frustrating dilemmas many of us face.

WEIGHT GAIN IS A SYMPTOM OF PCOS

Weight gain really is a symptom of PCOS, and you're not going mad if you've been trying to lose weight and finding it hard to shift those stubborn pounds. Research[2] shows that obesity is four times more likely in women who have PCOS and irregular periods than those without, simply because our metabolisms are wired differently.

Women with PCOS store fat more efficiently and burn up calories more slowly than women who don't have PCOS. According to PCOS expert Dr Helen Mason:

'Research has shown that overweight women with PCOS tend to eat less calories than women without, but they still struggle to lose weight. Even women with PCOS who are normal weight consider maintaining a normal weight as difficult a problem as those women who were over-weight, showing that the issue of weight is a constant struggle for everyone.'

This is borne out by a study[3] at the University of Pittsburgh where the diet of women with PCOS was compared with that of women who didn't have PCOS. The study found that although women with PCOS tended to be more overweight, there was virtually no difference in the two groups' dietary intake. But when lean women with PCOS were compared to lean women without PCOS, the investigators found that the former group consumed fewer calories to maintain their weight compared to their lean women who didn't have PCOS.

Why are we so 'efficient' at converting calories into fat? Or maintaining our weight with fewer calories? Here's the latest thinking:

THRIFTY GENES

Recent research[4] suggests that PCOS may be the result of 'thrifty' genes, providing advantages in times of food shortage. If you have 'thrifty' genes, you're very adept at storing calories for the famine that never comes.

HORMONES AND YOUR APPETITE

Other research has shown that the complex interplay of signalling proteins and hormones that regulate appetite is disrupted and disordered in PCOS, and this may trigger weight gain.

Leptin, a hormone produced by your fat cells, is involved in long-term weight and appetite regulation. It signals the hypothalamus gland in your brain when fat cells are full. Leptin levels should be in a balance, not too high and not too low. Low levels can result in food cravings.

If low leptin stimulates eating, you'd think that high leptin levels would inhibit eating. But this isn't the case, especially with overweight individuals. Overweight women with PCOS tend to have higher leptin levels than lean women,[5] but that doesn't stop them from eating. Therefore, it's thought that seriously overweight women may become resistant to the effects of leptin, and despite higher circulating levels of the hormone, don't experience its beneficial effects.[6] A diet high in saturated fats and low in fibre may contribute to leptin resistance.

Another hormone involved in appetite is ghrelin. A lot of research is being done on ghrelin right now, and we'll probably be hearing more about it in the years ahead. Ghrelin helps to regulate how much food you eat and how much weight you gain. In normal individuals ghrelin levels go up before meals, and down after meals. Elevated ghrelin triggers strong feelings of hunger. In addition to regulating eating, ghrelin may slow your metabolism and reduce your ability to burn fat.

Several studies[7] suggest that women with PCOS have disordered ghrelin levels, or an impaired ability to regulate ghrelin. One study showed that PCOS women were less satiated (less full, or 'satisfied') and their ghrelin levels didn't decline so much after a meal.

Cholecystokinin (CCK) is a hormone secreted in the gastrointestinal tract when you eat a meal. It slows down the digestive process and functions as a short-term satiety signal to inhibit food intake. But some women with PCOS have reduced CCK secretion after a meal, and this may play a role in the greater frequency of binge-eating and overweight in women with PCOS.[8]

The size and composition of your meals will influence ghrelin and leptin levels, and since the caloric size of your meal is partly determined by CCK, CCK in turn influences insulin and leptin. In short, we have a web of interconnecting hormones all influencing one thing: your metabolism.

A SLUGGISH METABOLISM

Your metabolic rate is the rate at which your body burns calories. The faster your metabolic rate, the more you can eat without putting on weight. The slower your metabolic rate, the more you need to watch your food intake.

Energy-use after a meal is called *postprandial thermogenesis*. For most people, postprandial thermogenesis accounts for a good percentage of their calorie burning (you can often see someone's speeded-up metabolism as they burn energy to digest their food if they get a red face or raised temperature after a meal), but studies[9] show that postprandial thermogenesis in women with PCOS is significantly reduced. Whether this is caused by leptin, ghrelin, insulin, CCK or a combination of all of them, the harsh truth is that if you have PCOS, you don't burn up as many calories after you eat a meal as someone who doesn't have PCOS. And the result is that you store more of the calories from the food you eat, which pushes up the likelihood of weight gain.

INSULIN RESISTANCE

If you've got insulin resistance as well as PCOS, you also have to deal with the consequence of insulin preventing you from burning calories off. Insulin resistance causes your body's hormones to react in the opposite way to what you really want – that is, to store energy as fat rather than burn it off.[10]

According to Dr Legro in the *American Journal of Obstetrics and Gynecology*, women with PCOS show as much as a 40 per cent lower response to the hormones that trigger the breakdown of fats than healthy women, whether or not the women with PCOS were obese.

WORKING TWICE AS HARD

As you can see, overweight women with PCOS tend to have multiple hormone disorders and genetic tendencies that predispose them to be overweight. So we do have to do more than the average person to control our weight. But the basics remain the same – you need to burn more calories than you take in.

Studies[11] show that at least 50 per cent of women with PCOS are overweight or obese. With the odds stacked against us, it's small wonder that many of us comfort eat or develop eating disorders, but the havoc eating disorders can wreak on your health will eventually make your symptoms worse.

▷ THE GOOD NEWS

Losing weight can be frustrating if you've got PCOS, but it's by no means impossible. The first essential step is to eat a healthy, balanced diet to help balance blood sugar and hormones, speed up your metabolism and reduce food cravings. The next step is to start doing things on top of your basic diet, exercise programme and lifestyle detox to help you lose weight. Some of the most effective ways for women with PCOS to lose weight – and keep it off – are listed below.

PORTION CONTROL

One of the healthiest ways to cut back on the calories without skimping on the nutrients is portion control. You don't need to cut out your favourite dishes, you just need to eat a little less of them. If you think that smaller portions won't satisfy your hunger, there are things you can do to give you that full feeling:

- Take time over your meals. Put your knife and fork down after each mouthful and chew food slowly.

- If you think you want to eat more, wait 10 or 15 minutes to see if you're still hungry. It takes a bit of time a while for your brain to recognize when your stomach is full.
- Never shop or cook when you're hungry. Keep a supply of healthy, low-fat, low-sugar snacks nearby, such as apple and nuts, dried fruit and low-fat yoghurt, so you never get really hungry.
- It takes time for your stomach to adjust to smaller portion size, so give yourself time and make sure you follow the 'little and often' rule. Around six meals a day is best for losing weight and for keeping hunger at bay. If there's a long gap between meals, blood sugar levels fall too low – leaving you tired, craving sugar and lacking in energy and concentration. Give your body food every few hours to boost your metabolic rate and keep blood sugar levels stable.
- Don't eat for several hours before you go to bed, say no later than 8 p.m. A light snack (say a cracker and a glass of low-fat milk) is OK, but not a heavy meal. It doesn't make sense to eat lots of food when all you're going to do is sleep. The earlier in the day you eat, the more likely you are to burn off the calories.
- Make nutrient-rich foods such as whole grains, fruits and vegetables the staples of your diet. They're filling but low in calories.

'It sounds ridiculous, but I went out and bought a set of smaller plates! Now I feel I'm getting a good plate of food, but it's less than before.'
Kerry, 29

BEAT FOOD CRAVINGS

Many women with PCOS find that they have strong sugar and carbohydrate cravings, and this plays havoc with their weight loss plans. We crave these foods because they send blood sugar levels rocketing, giving us an instant energy boost, but the boost is short lived as it leads to an overproduction of insulin followed by a dip in blood sugar, leaving us tired and craving the foods all over again.

If you suffer from food cravings, the healthy eating tips listed on pages 188–9 will help keep them at bay – but you can help yourself even more by using the glycaemic index when making your carbohydrate food choices. If you want to eat a food with a high GI, make sure you balance it with some protein and fat to slow down the release of sugar.

If your food cravings lead to food binges and comfort eating, you aren't alone: as many as 75 per cent of women who have weight to lose struggle with binge eating. If binges happen several times a week and you feel out of control, you probably have binge-eating disorder. If you suspect you have this you need to address this disorder separately from your efforts to lose weight. The best people to seek advice and help from are your doctor, a counsellor and a registered dietician. They will help you get your binges under control, and once you're better able to manage the bingeing you can look forward to real success with weight loss.

'Having a stock of healthy snacks in the fridge and a fruit bowl on my desk helps me eat something good instead of sugar.'
Debbie, 32

CHANGE YOUR HABITS

Small changes can add to up to big weight-loss results. Focus on a typical week and think of five things you could do differently that would help you cut back on calories. Here are some suggestions:

- Change your favourite snack. If you love ice cream and always have a bowl in the evening, try a different, healthier ice cream – look for low-fat low-sugar brands or frozen yoghurt that you can eat instead with some fruit. You could also cut down on your portion size.
- Instead of eating bread with a meal, have a glass of water and a handful of nuts before you sit down to eat. This will help fill your stomach and make you feel more full.
- If you normally grab a packet of crisps as you watch TV, don't give them up altogether. Instead, take out a handful, seal up the bag and put it away. Then enjoy your serving of crisps slowly.
- If you go out with your friends every weekend and everyone orders a pizza, make the decision to order your own personal-size pizza. Better yet, just eat half and take the rest home for a quick lunch the next day. Skip the beer and order a diet soda instead. Swap a large latte for a regular. Find a healthy way to have fun with your friends and make it your new routine – try a dance class or a bike ride.

'I used to grab breakfast and gulp it down standing up. Sitting down to eat makes me take time so I feel fuller quicker!'
Catherine, 41

NATURAL DIET BOOSTERS

- Eating regularly, say three main meals and three snacks a day, is crucial. 'Don't skip breakfast,' says Marilyn Glenville, a nutritional therapist and author of *Natural Alternatives to Dieting*. 'Eating breakfast fires up your metabolism so that you end up burning more calories. Make sure you eat regularly, as this gives your body the message that there's a plentiful supply of food, so that there's no need for it to store food.'

- A good night's sleep is important, too, as lack of sleep disrupts hormones, triggering changes in metabolism so that you're not processing food as well as you should. It's thought that lack of sleep is linked with higher levels of cortisol, which can throw your metabolism out of balance. Other studies[12] have shown it can have a negative effect on carbohydrate metabolism and endocrine function, lowering glucose tolerance and making it more difficult to convert carbohydrates into energy. This makes it more likely that fats and sugars are stored as unwanted extra pounds. Other research has established a link between lack of sleep and increased appetite, largely because cortisol is important in appetite control.

- Drinking four cups of green tea each day is said to help you lose weight. Studies at the American Society for Clinical Nutrition found that one of its compounds, catechol, increases metabolism and reduces the amount of fat your body absorbs by as much as 30 per cent. Green tea is rich in natural antioxidants which fight the damaging effects of free radicals.

- Drinking a glass of water before you eat can aid weight loss because you feel fuller. Water helps to flush out toxins and waste, and fat can be broken down only in the presence of water. Water can also have a direct impact on energy – we may reach for a sugar fix when what we need to do is rehydrate the body.

- Research has shown that eating chillies or hot peppers can boost your metabolism and reduce your appetite. A study in Melbourne found that volunteers who added red pepper to their diet ate fewer calories. 'They whiz up your metabolic rate by a hefty 25 per cent,' says Dr Caroline Shreeve, author of *Fat-burning Foods*. 'Chilli, cayenne and pepper and mustard should all hit the spot.'

- Cinnamon contains substances which can help the body convert sugar into energy so it's less likely to be stored as fat.

- Scientists in San Diego, California claim you can lose almost a pound a month by adding grapefruit to your usual meals. They monitored 100 overweight volunteers, asking a third to eat half a grapefruit before a meal, a third to drink a glass of grapefruit juice, and the other third to avoid grapefruit. After 12 weeks the grapefruit group has lost an average of 3.6 pounds, the juice group 3.3 pounds and the last group nothing. 'Including grapefruit in your diet can be really helpful,' says Marilyn Glenville. 'Grapefruit reduces insulin levels, which in turn leads to a reduction in the amount of body fat stores.' But Marilyn warns 'If you're on medication check with your doctor first, as grapefruit can slow the drugs being metabolized by your system and can make a medication more concentrated.'

- Having a bowl of soup may also help you lose weight. US researchers at Johns Hopkins University in Baltimore found that people who chose soup as a starter consumed 25 per cent less fat in the following main meal than those who chose a high-fat dessert.

- Acupuncture, properly applied, removes hunger pangs by stimulating the release of the so-called pleasure hormones, endorphins, which are stimulated by food. Because acupuncture does the work of food in this way, your stomach doesn't miss it and hunger pangs don't occur. Moreover, specialists in acupuncture claim that the effects last even after the course of the acupuncture is over.

⇨ WEIGHT GAIN ISN'T ALWAYS DOWN TO PCOS

Take a look and see if any of the following apply to you.

- Your weight gain could be due to water retention – drink more water, cut down on salt.
- Many allergy sufferers find that anti-histamines increase their appetite. Not only that, but those with hayfever can also wake up hundreds of times each night, a problem known as 'microarousal', leaving you feeling exhausted and more likely to eat comfort foods for energy.
- Are you guilty of e-mailing your colleagues instead of walking over to speak to them face to face? If so, you're likely to gain 1lb a year.
- There's some preliminary evidence[13] suggesting that artificial sweeteners can play tricks on your body's natural ability to count calories, so be mindful of that if you find yourself using a lot of artificial sweetener.
- Drinks high in fructose can suppress appetite-regulating chemicals in our bodies. So you're better off eating whole fruit and having herbal teas.
- A lot of so-called low-fat and fat-free foods are packaged, processed and offer reduced calories, but not much else in terms of nutrition – in fact low-fat often means high-sugar. The exceptions: low-fat yoghurt, low-fat cheese and low-fat milk, which can provide some nutrients.
- Chronic stress increases cortisol, which is a stress-response hormone.

Elevated cortisol is associated with insulin resistance and increased abdominal fat. A great reason to book that relaxing massage! (We've got plenty of advice on how to reduce stress in Part 3.)

- We've mentioned this many times before, but it's so important we just have to mention it again. Every time you eat, your metabolic rate speeds up by 20–30 per cent for the next two hours, but if you skip meals you miss out on this. Missing breakfast is the biggest problem – your metabolic rate slows by 5 per cent overnight, and stays at this rate until you next eat.

- The liver is the main fat-burning organ of the body, but if it's overloaded with toxins such as alcohol, it's too busy handling these to process fat effectively. So cut down on the booze, refined sugar and saturated fat.

- Fast-food salads can contain more calories than a burger. A McDonald's chicken caesar salad with dressing has 452 calories, compared to a McChicken sandwich, with just 375. If you want to eat fast food now and again, it pays to do your research.

- Both yoga and Pilates increase muscle tone and condition, but to really burn calories you need to combine them with some aerobic work.

- Experts at Tulane University in the US have discovered that heart rate, blood pressure and metabolic rate slow so much while we watch TV that we burn 20–30 calories an hour less than if we simply sat still. Turn it off!

- Be warned: most brown bread is as refined as white bread. Choose granary, wholegrain or seeded breads because they take longer for the body to digest and don't trigger insulin surges.

- A large proportion of PCOS women have thyroid dysfunction, resulting in a lower metabolic rate and great difficulty in losing weight. If you're tired all the time, gaining weight and really feeling the cold, then your thyroid could be sluggish, which in turn slows down your metabolism. Combat it by upping your intake of 'good' fats like oily fish and nuts.

WEIGHT-LOSS SUPPLEMENTS

If you're deficient in certain nutrients this could hinder your weight-loss plans. The major weight-loss supplements available for women with PCOS are listed below – but once again, remember that they can only be effective if you follow a healthy diet as well. (For more details on these, see page 147.)

- B vitamins – help you to control fat metabolism and digest your food
- Chromium – needed to help insulin control blood sugar levels. May also help control levels of fat and cholesterol in the blood.
- Manganese – helps with the absorption of fats and also works to stabilize blood sugar levels.
- Magnesium – aids in the production of insulin
- Co-enzyme Q10 – needed for energy production, and can help with weight loss
- Zinc – can help control appetite

Other nutritional supplements recommended for weight loss include potassium and calcium (which, like zinc, are important in the production of energy), EFAs for appetite control, psyllium husks for fibre, mineral-rich kelp, lecithin capsules which can help break down fat, spirulina which can help stabilize blood sugar, vitamin C to speed up a slow metabolism, boron to speed up the burning of calories (raisons and onions are good sources) and the amino acids L-Ornithine, L-Arginine and L-lysine, as research has shown that weight loss can be improved with a combination of these. We mention them in case your doctor, dietician or nutritional therapist suggests them.

Apart from your daily multivitamin and –mineral, if you want to take any supplements you should consult your doctor or a nutritional therapist.

If you want to take any herbal or fat-fighting supplements to help you lose weight, such as Siberian ginseng, *Garcinia cambogia*, fennel or fenugreek, the same applies. Certain herbal supplements can be toxic in large doses. Ephedra is a popular ingredient in many over-the-counter weight loss formulations, but it has been shown to cause irregular heartbeats, strokes, hypertension and anxiety – hardly a harmless profile, so best avoided. Unless your doctor feels that your weight poses a serious risk to your health, steer clear of slimming drugs of any kind. What you need is permanent weight loss: the drawback of slimming drugs is that they are like fad diets: they don't work in the long term. The best way to lose weight is to gain control of your eating habits and increase the amount of exercise you get, for life.

A REGISTERED DIETICIAN

If you and your doctor are very concerned about your weight, you may want to enlist the support of a registered dietician or nutritionist. Dieticians can be a great source of support and insight. They can help you understand why you aren't losing weight and support you in your new programme. These professionals have studied good nutrition and can save you a lot of time and experimentation on your own.

Ideally you should also ask your doctor to refer you to a dietician who is experienced with women with PCOS. If you've been diagnosed with insulin resistance, a dietician who specializes in diabetes may be just what you need.

SURGERY

Bariatric surgery for weight loss is a radical but increasingly popular form of weight management. There are many variations, but the basic principle is to change the way the stomach receives food. For example, the actual size of the stomach may be reduced. Another method may be to bypass parts of the intestine or to wire the jaws so that the person can take in only small amounts of food.

These drastic methods, along with medically-supervised ketosis (extreme high protein starvation diet), are intended only for the seriously overweight who have exhausted all other options. For the great majority of women with PCOS, these methods won't be needed.

▷ BMI AND WAIST-TO-HIP RATIO

The BMI is a formula that is better at predicting the risk of disease than body weight alone. If you want to know your BMI, multiply your weight in pounds by 700, then divide the product by your height in inches squared. If the result is between 19 and 25, you're at a healthy weight. A number of 27 or higher is an indication that you're overweight.

Do take into account your body shape when setting your weight loss goals. Apple and pear shapes are definitely not equal when it comes to the risk of developing diabetes. If you're an apple, the risk is higher.

LOSE WEIGHT GRADUALLY!

Making diet and lifestyle changes according to the guidelines in this chapter, and the previous three, is the most successful way to lose weight – but it takes time (typically a good three to six months) before you see the benefits.

If weight loss isn't immediate it can be tempting to restrict calories, but this never works in the long term as it slows down your metabolism. The only way to lose weight safely and to keep it off for the long term is to change your eating habits and exercise regularly.

You should aim to lose no more than two pounds a week. It may seem slow, but the important thing is that this steady approach to weight loss works.

BOOST YOUR MOTIVATION

Losing weight isn't easy under any circumstances, but if you've got PCOS there's even more dieting stress than normal, so motivation is critical. It's all very well saying 'I need to watch my weight' but it's easy to get bored or put things off. So if you're reading this book and still can't get motivated, we hope the following tips will help:

- Keep a food diary. This helps you think about whether your diet is helping your symptoms or making them worse. A food diary gives you a feeling of control – but the most important thing about writing down what you eat is the awareness it brings and the way it encourages you to notice what you're doing. You can't change habits you aren't aware of.

- 'Diet with a friend who's got PCOS too so you can keep each other on track, share recipes and dieting tips.' says Sandra, 28. PCOS support groups are good places to find a weight-loss buddy.

- Do it for yourself first – to improve the quality of your health and your life, to more easily do an activity that you like and to feel better when you try on new clothes.

- If you go off your new eating habits for an evening or a weekend, don't quit. Just pick up where you left off. Remember the 80/20 rule.

- Find ways to reward yourself. Keep it simple and inexpensive, but if you meet a weight-loss goal buy yourself a new pair of earrings or have a long bath with the door locked. Whatever you decide to do, make sure you find time to celebrate your success.

- Throw away the bathroom scales. Instead, monitor yourself by the way your clothes fit and the way you look and feel.

- Draw up a contract with yourself to change your eating and exercise routines in ways that can help you become slimmer and fitter. A contract with yourself may sound odd, but research shows that writing down your goals and aspirations makes them more real and helps you stay focused on achieving them.

- Motivational techniques such as visualization can help you get in touch with what you really want. Close your eyes and imagine yourself 20 years older. In all those 20 years you haven't made any healthy changes to your lifestyle. Now imagine what you'd look like. Such techniques can be shocking, but they can bring focus and commitment to your weight-loss plan.

- Learn all you can about the huge benefits of weight loss for women with PCOS. Weight loss can not only manage your day-to-day symptoms but can also reduce your risk of poor health in the future. Thinking of these benefits can be a powerful way to keep you going.
- Think about all the benefits you'll personally gain when you lose weight. No matter how silly they appear, write them down. This will help you see up front what you stand to gain if you start taking steps to manage your weight. Let this list motivate you, re-energize you and keep you going.

'When I feel myself trying to make excuses for not going to the gym, I think about all the other things exercise brings me, not just about how I need to lose weight. I get clearer skin, diabetes protection and time to just think my own thoughts and listen to some music.'
Emma-Jane, 39

KEEP YOUR COOL

Above all, don't stress yourself about losing weight. Instead, spend your energy motivating yourself to eat healthily and exercise regularly, not just for a few weeks but for the rest of your life. If you're focused on good health and follow the advice in this book, natural weight loss, along with a reduction in your symptoms, will almost certainly follow.

'It took me ages to stop being obsessed with losing loads of weight really quickly. But the thing that made me slow down was looking at old photo albums. I could see that over the years I'd yo-yo'd, and that all the crash diets I'd been on hadn't helped me keep the weight off in the long term. I still do get impatient, but when I do, I look at those pictures again and it really helps.'

Sarah, 43

'I've decided to forget about losing weight. I'm a size 18 and only 5' 4 so I need to lose some. But I'm hoping this will just be a side-effect of my healthier new lifestyle.'

Karen, 29

CHAPTER 12
FERTILITY-BOOSTING SECRETS THAT WORK

If fertility is a concern for you, you're certainly not alone. It's estimated that as many as 80 per cent of women with PCOS have a problem with fertility. Research[1] shows that women with PCOS are more concerned about their fertility than women without, and that this can affect their quality of life.

When your periods are absent or irregular, there are often problems with ovulation. Without an egg in the right place at the right time to receive a sperm, you can't get pregnant. And even if you do, the incidence of miscarriage for women with PCOS is thought to be higher than average.[2] But don't panic. There's plenty of good news.

Research[3] shows that many women with PCOS get pregnant and give birth to healthy babies readily, once they get their symptoms under control by balancing underlying hormone levels. And in many cases these pregnancies occur without fertility drugs – over 70 per cent of women with PCOS do manage to conceive naturally in the end. Over 20 per cent manage to conceive with treatment.

Expert in reproductive endocrinology Dr Samuel Thatcher says, 'Therapy may be as much 90 per cent effective of fertility problems related to PCOS.' So how can you help maximize your chances of fertility? This chapter is packed with practical ideas.

WHAT'S CAUSING THE PROBLEM?

As we've seen, PCOS is a metabolic disorder that triggers a series of hormonal imbalances, including raised testosterone and potential insulin resistance, all of which can stop you ovulating and getting pregnant. But these symptoms don't mean you're infertile. Infertility means not being able to have a baby when you want one, and 70 per cent of PCOS sufferers can conceive naturally. If you've got PCOS and have absent or irregular periods or problems with ovulation, you're not infertile – you have a condition known as subfertility. This means that getting pregnant may not be as simple for you as it is for some women, but it's by no means impossible.

'Don't let anyone tell you you're infertile or can't have children. You need to have proper tests, not just accept a diagnosis of infertility along with PCOS.' **Deanne, 27**

If you can bring your hormones back into a more regular pattern with healthy diet and lifestyle changes you can increase your chances of getting pregnant. This isn't to say that you can get pregnant overnight if you eat well and lose weight. After all, even 'normal' couples are expected to try for a year before undergoing any medical investigation.

And even though PCOS is one of the leading causes of fertility problems, there are other factors you need to bear in mind. For example, over 40 per cent of problems with fertility are related to inadequate sperm quality, function or motility. Your doctor may also want to rule out uterine or cervical abnormalities, fibroid tumours, blocked fallopian tubes, endometriosis and/or pelvic adhesions. There's also 'unexplained infertility' that remains undefined in spite of an extensive medical evaluation. So even though your primary concern is about ovarian problems, you shouldn't be afraid to ask your doctor to rule out other causes, especially if you've been trying for 12 months.

▷ HOW LONG WILL YOU BE FERTILE?

A new test has been launched in January 2006 that promises to help women plan when to have children by indicating how many eggs are left in their ovaries. The 'Plan Ahead' test works by measuring the levels of three hormones in blood, taken from the arm, on the second or third day of a woman's cycle. After posting the sample off to the laboratory of Lifestyle Choices, which has launched the test, the woman receives an analysis of the number of eggs remaining in the ovaries compared with the average population at that age. The woman's ovarian reserve for the following two years can also be forecast, helping her to decide whether she should risk delaying trying for a baby. The test was developed by Professor Bill Ledger from the University of Sheffield, who hopes the test will 'help many women avoid the anguish caused by the early or unexpected arrival of declining fertility and menopause'.

PRECONCEPTUAL CARE

Getting pregnant isn't just about having lots of sex. Research[4] shows that everything you do in the three or four months before trying to conceive can be as important as the sex itself. What you drink, eat, breathe, do as a job, how stressed you are, how you feel about yourself – everything matters.

There's a lot you can do to prepare your body for a healthy pregnancy, and the good news is that the self-help approach has helped countless women with PCOS get pregnant and have healthy babies.

Research[5] on women with PCOS has shown how effective diet and lifestyle change can be for reducing weight, acne, irregular periods and facial hair, and increasing the chances of natural conception and a healthy full-term pregnancy.

In an ideal world we'd recommend that you follow this plan for three to four months before trying to conceive to maximize your chances of a healthy pregnancy. This is because it takes about three months for a new batch of sperm to be made, and three months for a woman's egg to develop from its follicle and be released. It also takes about three months to eliminate certain fertility-limiting toxins from your system properly and raise the level of crucial fertility-boosting nutrients in your blood serum.[6]

Taking care of yourself before you want to get pregnant won't just boost your fertility, it's crucial for your baby, too. The egg that is released at conception is the product of your diet and lifestyle, and experts[7] now believe that what a woman eats prior to conception is just as significant to the health of the baby as what she eats during pregnancy. According to Irwin Emanuel, MD, Professor of Epidemiology and Pediatrics at the University of Seattle, 'If you're undernourished your baby could become programmed at conception to develop high blood pressure, clotting disorders, abnormal glucose, insulin and cholesterol problems and even hormonal problems like PCOS.'

IT TAKES TWO

Every one of us is different and there's no magic formula that will work for us all, but healthy diet and lifestyle choices for you and your partner before you get pregnant can yield dramatic results. Never lose sight of the fact that getting pregnant takes two, and your partner can help to boost his own fertility at the same time as you are enhancing yours.

For men the most common problem is sperm quality. In other words is the sperm strong and fit enough to reach and penetrate a ripe egg?

Both sperm quality and quantity can be affected by lifestyle factors such as poor diet, stress, weight gain, too little exercise, smoking and alcohol. In addition, your partner should avoid hot baths, tight underpants, and exposure to heat, traffic fumes, mobile phones and long hours sitting and driving. Knowing this gives a man a great deal of control over his own fertility, and numerous studies have shown that simple diet and lifestyle changes can improve sperm in as little as three months.[8] So it's the best idea for you both to follow the action plan over the page.

'It felt great when we both decided to get healthier together. We feel like a team and we encourage each other.'
Sarah, 29

YOUR 5-POINT FERTILITY BOOSTING ACTION PLAN

I: MANAGE YOUR WEIGHT

Carrying too much body fat can make symptoms of PCOS – including irregular periods – worse and stop you getting pregnant. Losing weight, if you have weight to lose, can improve your symptoms and boost your fertility.

We know that both PCOS and obesity increase the risk of infertility, but thankfully the effect is quickly reversed. Research[9] has shown that losing even a small amount of weight can be enough to stimulate ovulation and make periods regular. Follow our weight-management guidelines in the previous chapter and remember that the best way to lose weight isn't to diet but simply to eat healthily and increase the amount you exercise.

If weight gain, not weight loss, is your goal, don't be tempted to reach for the biscuits and junk food. Aim to eat little and often and to eat plenty of healthy, fresh foods, full of fertility-boosting goodness.

2. GET AS FIT AND WELL AS YOU CAN

Becoming as fit and as well as you can involves you and your partner exercising regularly as well as getting the all-clear from your doctor and getting checked and treated for any infections.

Regular exercise can boost your fertility. Not only can it kick-start weight loss but it can also help insulin and glucose control, which in turn means your ovaries are encouraged to produce less testosterone, promote hormonal balance and ease symptoms. For tips on how to get started with exercise and fit it into your daily life, refer to Chapter 7.

As well as eating healthily and exercising regularly, you and your partner also need to find a qualified, experienced physician to work with to ensure you are both as fit as you can possibly be. You will need to be thoroughly evaluated to determine the probable causes of your infertility, and what can be done about it. The doctor should do a complete medical history, physical examinations as indicated, and laboratory testing as indicated by your health status, physical findings and medical history.

▷ **HOW OLD ARE YOU?**

Are you over 35? Although more and more women are having babies later in life, it's important to bear in mind that the twenties are considered to be the reproductive prime, with the least amount of fertility and health complications for mother and child. Whether you have PCOS or not, at about the age of 35 most women start to get less fertile and may not ovulate every month. If you have PCOS and are having problems conceiving, clearly being over 35 isn't going to boost your chances, but try not to let this panic you. Recent research[10] has suggested that older women aren't the only ones prone to having defective eggs – young women have flaws in about half of theirs, too. Whatever your age, you can raise your fertility levels with diet, exercise, healthy checks and, if needed, fertility treatment. There's a lot you can do to help yourself.

In the preconception period you will also need to use a form of contraception you can trust, but which will also allow your fertility to return quickly when you stop using it. You need to discuss what options are available with your doctor. More research needs to be done, but the indications are that the combined pill carries with it a risk of a delay of a year or more in conceiving once you come off it. Barrier methods of birth control (diaphragm, cap, condom) are probably your best choice as they don't involve hormonal manipulation, and your fertility will return as soon as you stop using them.

Natural family planning – learning to recognize what time of the month you're fertile – seems to work for some couples, but it isn't foolproof even for women with regular cycles. If you've got irregular or absent cycles, as many women with PCOS have, natural family planning isn't a good choice.

3. DE-STRESS

Find ways to deal with stress. Chronic stress increases cortisol, a stress-response hormone, and elevated cortisol is associated with insulin resistance, excess testosterone and increased abdominal fat, all of which can make your symptoms worse and reduce fertility.

Studies[11] show that both emotional and physical stress can stop women ovulating. And stress can influence a man's libido as well as his sperm. Progressive fertility units such as the Beth Israel Hospital in Boston, US and the Harvard Behaviour Medicine Program have been including stress reduction in their fertility-boosting programmes for years. 'Our experience at the Division of Behavior Medicine in the Beth Israel Deaconess Center (and this is backed up with research)[12] is that women with long-term infertility may well increase their chances of conception when they reduce their levels of stress,' says Alice Domar, Director of the Mind/Body Institute at the Center.

An International European Survey[13] has identified stressful work as a major risk factor in infertility, but whatever the reason for your stress – be it anxiety about PCOS or worries about paying the bills, or because of troubles in your relationship – you may find that this interferes with your health and your fertility. In the same way that a poor diet can stop you ovulating, emotional stress has been shown to suppress ovulation and menstrual cycle function.

It's also important to point out that stress can trigger loss of libido – and if you're not enjoying sex or having much of it, obviously you're less likely to get pregnant. Stress is a fact of life so you can't avoid it, but you can find ways to manage it and help influence your body to conceive. Start with the ideas in Chapter 15.

4. EAT FRESH HEALTHY FOOD

You can improve your fertility by what you eat. Dr Margaret Rayman, Director of the MSc Course in Nutrition Medicine at the University of Surrey, says:

> 'The food you eat affects every single cell and system in your entire body and is needed to produce healthy eggs and sperm for the development of your baby when you get pregnant. A healthy balanced diet in the preconceptual period will not only boost your chances of having a healthy baby, it will keep your weight down and your blood sugar levels in balance. If your blood sugar levels aren't balanced, then your hormones, which control your fertility, won't work properly either.'

As we've seen, healthy eating according to our PCOS diet guidelines in Chapter 6 can restore your blood sugar and hormone balance, improve your energy levels and help you lose weight, as well as addressing irregular periods and infertility. A healthy, balanced diet will help you include enough of the important baby-making minerals:

- Iron – find it in eggs, fish, dark green vegetables, lean red meat, and pulses, dark chocolate, dried apricots and Guinness!
- Zinc – get your full share (about 15mg a day) by eating lean turkey, chicken, almonds, beans, wheatgerm, yoghurt, oatmeal, corn, eggs, and whole grains
- Magnesium – good sources include nuts, vegetables, brown rice and sunflower seeds
- Selenium – include some nuts in your diet, as selenium deficiency can reduce your egg production. Brazil and cashew nuts are particularly good.

In addition to these don't forget to get your fill of vitamin B_6, vitamin C, vitamin E, folic acid and essential fats (EFAs). Several studies have shown that B_6 is essential for hormone balance and fertility in women (wild pink yams, lentils and watermelons are particularly good sources). Vitamin C can help trigger ovulation and, along with vitamin E, it may help preserve fertility for longer. Vitamin C is found in raw fruits and vegetables, particularly berries and green sprouting vegetables like Brussels sprouts. Vitamin E food sources include wheatgerm, seeds, nuts, oily fish and broccoli. Folic acid won't make you fertile but it's critical to your baby's health – not just in the earliest days of pregnancy but before you even conceive. You'll find folic acid in spinach and other green leafy veg, citrus fruits, nuts, legumes and enriched products such as grains, and it's essential to take a good supplement throughout pregnancy. Essential fats are found in nuts, seeds and oily fish.

Your partner needs to eat a wide range of nutrients, too. Research has shown that the following nutrients are of special importance to men because of their impact on sperm quality: vitamin A, B complex, magnesium, calcium, selenium, vitamin E, folic acid and manganese.

Taking a good daily multivitamin and -mineral is a good idea. According to researchers[14] from the University of Leeds it may double your chances of getting pregnant and help you produce better quality eggs.

Too much soya isn't a good idea if you're trying to get pregnant, as a study by King's College London in early 2005 found that a compound in soya called genistein could stop sperm reaching the egg, thus decreasing fertility. Limit to no more than five or six small portions of soy a week.

'If nothing else, eating well helped me feel more energized, happier and able to cope with stress. And it seems madness not to do my best when Sheila is doing hers.'

Anthony, 34

5. DETOX YOUR LIFESTYLE

You've probably been exposed to all sorts of petrochemicals, heavy metals and other toxins over your lifetime, from cigarette smoke to traffic fumes and pesticides and preservatives used on food. Some of these substances can act as hormone mimics or disrupters, and for women with PCOS this is bad news. Toxins can also affect the quality and quantity of your partner's sperm, so you could both benefit from a gentle detox.

To explore the issue of removing toxic substances from your body, see Chapter 8.

NATURAL THERAPIES FOR FERTILITY

From the many conversations, letters and e-mails we've had, it's clear that natural therapies have helped a significant number of women with PCOS have babies.

Researchers at the University of Surrey followed 367 couples for 3 years. Some 37 per cent of these couples had a history of infertility, and 38 per cent of the women had had previous miscarriages. They were put on a programme consisting of organic foods, an individualized vitamin supplement, and alcohol and tobacco avoidance. At the end of the study, 89 per cent of the couples had given birth to healthy babies, and none had a miscarriage. Although this study[15] was preliminary, it does suggest that a healthy diet and lifestyle increase the probability of pregnancy and reduce the chances of miscarriage.

There aren't many specific studies about natural therapies for PCOS or their impact on fertility. However, many women with PCOS say that certain safe, non-toxic and effective natural therapies have helped restore menstrual function and ovulation. The therapies women with PCOS have considered helpful are outlined below.

NUTRITIONAL THERAPY PLUS LIFESTYLE CHANGE

On top of lifestyle changes and healthy eating recommendations, a nutritional therapist can help you work out which specific nutrients you may be lacking and help you work out a programme of diet and supplements uniquely tailored to you and your lifestyle.

Much of the advice given by a nutritional therapist will be the same as the advice given in the PCOS fertility-boosting action plan. You've seen how important preconceptual care is, and you've also seen how healthy lifestyle recommendations and certain supplements have scientific backing. For example, studies show that weight management has been shown to help women with PCOS conceive; certain nutrients such as B_6 are linked to increased fertility; and taking a daily multivitamin and -mineral can boost your fertility and your chances of success if you're undergoing assisted conception. Of all the natural therapies you might like to explore, a healthy diet and lifestyle changes are the most sensible and the most helpful, especially because you can take charge yourself.

Note:

When taking any kind of supplement always seek advice from a dietician, doctor or nutritional therapist.

HERBAL MEDICINE

Herbalism is a very popular choice for women with PCOS and has shown some promising results. Many herbs are natural forms of medicine that have been used for generations, and a herbalist can help to regulate periods and boost fertility.

There's more research evidence available regarding Chinese herbal medicine than there is for Western medical herbalism, but the herb *Agnus castus* has been shown to be effective in correcting hormonal imbalances.

For more detailed information see Chapter 9.

REFLEXOLOGY

This therapy is gaining a cult status among women with PCOS as a great way to boost chances of pregnancy. There has even been a little research done – a small trial in Denmark examined 108 women with an average age of 30 who had been trying to conceive for an average of 6.7 years. Many dropped out of the trial, but 19 of the remaining 61 conceived within six months of completing the treatment.

Reflexologists Frances Box and Jacqui Garnier both work in the UK, specializing in fertility issues and PCOS respectively, with impressive results. Working on the parts of the foot corresponding to the pituitary gland, which controls the flow of hormones, Box also uses aromatherapy on patients with fertility problems to alleviate stress. Ask other women you know with PCOS if they can recommend someone, or contact the National Reflexology Association (see Resources section).

ACUPUNCTURE

There's published evidence to show that acupuncture works for problems such as back pain, toothaches and migraines, and a clinical trial[16] published in *Gynecological Endocrinology* in 1992 suggests that acupuncture can help with infertility. The word among PCOS communities is that acupuncture can really help to kickstart non-existant periods or regularize irregular ones. According to a 2002 study, acupuncture timed with in-vitro fertilization increased conception rates. The group receiving acupuncture had a success rate of 43 per cent vs only 26 per cent for the control group.[17]

HYPNOTHERAPY

Subconscious worries can prevent conception, so hypnotherapy can deal with any doubts about your future role as a mother, says Julie Gerland, a clinical hypnotherapist and founder of the Centre of University Unity in Hong Kong. There was also some evidence published in the *European Journal of Clinical Hypnosis* in 1994, which stated that hypnotherapy could help in medically unexplained, functional and psychosomatic infertility.

> 'I was so anxious about whether I'd be a good mum, and what I'd do if I couldn't get pregnant, that having hypnotherapy really helped.'
> **Janice, 33**

HOMOEOPATHY

In a 2000 German study,[18] 30 infertile women with hormonal problems were given homoeopathic remedies, while a matched group was treated with placebo. The results for the homoeopathic group were encouraging, and increasingly medical experts are suggesting homoeopathy as a complement or alternative to conventional medicine.

CONVENTIONAL FERTILITY TREATMENTS

Because most women with PCOS don't ovulate, the first conventional medical treatment option for infertility is usually the administration of drugs to induce ovulation.

- Clomiphene citrate (Brand names Clomid or Serophene) is taken for five days early in your cycle to stimulate ovulation. Clomid may not be effective if taken for more than six menstrual cycles. Research suggests that about two-thirds of women taking Clomid ovulate within four cycles, and some studies show that around 35 per cent achieve pregnancy. Unfortunately, many women with PCOS are Clomid resistant and don't ovulate even when taking the maximum dose. Recent studies, however, show that when taken with an insulin sensitizer such as metformin (see page 55), Clomid significantly increases the chances of ovulation and pregnancy.

- There's some evidence to suggest that Clomid may increase your risk of ovarian cancer if taken for 12 or more cycles. Clomid also has a number of side-effects including bowel problems, headache, dizziness, blurred vision and depression.

- hCG (human chorionic gonadotrophin) may be used in conjunction with Clomid. hCG has the same effect on the follicle as LH (luteinizing hormone): it stimulates the dominant follicle to release its egg. hCG is given by injection, and has to be carefully timed. If given too soon, ovulation may be blocked. Too much hCG may cause ovarian hyperstimulation and cyst formation.

- hMG (human menopausal gonadotrophin, most commonly known as Pergonal) is a combination of LH (luteinizing hormone) and FSH (follicle-stimulating hormone) derived from the urine of menopausal women. Both LH and FSH are required for follicle development. It's given by injection. Too much hMG may cause ovarian hyperstimulation and cyst formation, and there's also a risk of multiple pregnancy.

- FSH (follicle-stimulating hormone) is an injectable drug intended for women who already have enough LH. Since many women with PCOS have excessive LH, FSH can be helpful in some cases at triggering ovulation. Side-effects can include mood swings and hyperstimulation of the ovaries.

- GnRH is naturally released from your hypothalamus gland in pulses every 90 minutes. GnRH causes your pituitary gland to release both LH and FSH, which are necessary for follicle development. To mimic the 90-minute pulse, you will have to wear a pump 24 hours a day, which injects GnRH every 90 minutes. One benefit of GnRH is reduced risk of ovarian hyperstimulation or a multiple pregnancy. GnRH may be used when Clomid and gonadotrophin injections have failed.

There are still glaring gaps in our knowledge about the dangers and side-effects of fertility drugs, and some believe they may increase the risk of ovarian cancer.[19] The best advice we can give is to proceed with caution under the best advice from your healthcare practitioner, and using your own and your partner's knowledge and instincts about what's right for you.

If fertility-boosting drugs are unsuccessful, there are a number of medical interventions that may help you to get pregnant.

- Ovarian surgery – If other treatments have failed, surgery may be an option. It can't cure PCOS but it can promote ovulation to increase your chances of getting pregnant. Ovarian drilling is an outpatient laparoscopic procedure where a laser is used to pierce the thickened coat of the ovary, to drain fluid from it and trigger ovulation.
- IUI – intrauterine insemination. IUI is a medical procedure that places your partner's sperm directly into your uterus. The advantage of IUI is that it puts a much larger number of sperm into your uterus than

would occur normally with intercourse. IUI may be useful if your partner has a low sperm count. Assuming you're ovulating, a pregnancy success rate of about 15 per cent has been reported.

- IVF – in-vitro fertilization. IVF refers to removal of eggs from your body, fertilizing them with your partner's sperm and then implanting a fertilized egg into your womb. Although simple in concept, the execution of this procedure is complex – and expensive.

- GIFT – gamete intra-fallopian transfer. GIFT involves collection of eggs, mixing them with sperm, and placing a maximum of three fertilized eggs into your fallopian tubes. The eggs are obtained by a laparoscope inserted through the abdomen, so general anaesthesia may be required.

- ICSI – intracytoplasmic sperm injection. This procedure involves injecting a single sperm into a single egg. The technique isn't very successful in cases where the egg quality is poor. Another minor factor to consider is that there's no competition among sperm, where, under normal circumstances, the healthiest sperm would be the one that joins the egg. A team of Japanese scientists has suggested, after trials, that removal of the sperm's acrosome cap could improve the efficiency of this treatment.

In summary, the overall pregnancy success rate for IVF and embryo transfers is reported to be in the 25–50 per cent range, though there's a lot of individual variability.

Whatever method you choose to stay fertile or achieve pregnancy, one thing is certain: maintaining your health and well-being all the way through to motherhood is essential for increasing your chances of having a successful pregnancy and healthy baby. Fertility treatments can leave you feeling quite powerless, but healthy diet and lifestyle changes can enhance the power of any fertility treatment, boost your energy and give you a feeling of control.

All the same, if you're trying to get pregnant and can't, we hope the 'coping with anxiety' tips in Part 3 will help. We also recommend you find or create an infertility support group. A recent Harvard study[20] showed that women who participated in an infertility support group had a 25 per cent increase in their success rate over women who just got the usual infertility clinic care. An excellent resource for PCOS support groups is the Polycystic Ovarian Syndrome Association: www.pcosupport.org, and Verity in the UK (www.verity-pcos.org.uk).

YOUR HEALTHY PCOS PREGNANCY

As we saw in Chapter 4, the risk of miscarriage, gestational diabetes, unusually small or large babies and pregnancy-induced hypertension appears to increase in women with PCOS. Some of these risks are linked to pre-pregnancy weight and some to insulin resistance, while the smaller birthweight babies may be the result of alternations in the PCOS ovary itself. But don't panic – thousands of women with PCOS have successful pregnancies every year.

The increased risk of miscarriage in many women with PCOS may be due to a protein deficiency. Research is ongoing, but in 2005 scientists from the Monash Institute of Medical Research and Sydney's St Vincent Hospital found that women who suffered miscarriages were deficient in a protein called MIC1, which is responsible for healthy development of the life-giving placenta in the womb.

There is also a chance that breastfeeding may not come as easily to women with PCOS. More research is needed, but it's possible that the hormonal imbalances of PCOS have an inhibiting effect on prolactin, the hormone crucial to milk production.

Every pregnancy carries with it risks, whether you have PCOS or not, but do you need to see a specialist in prenatal medicine if you have PCOS? The jury is out, but most gynaecologists think probably not. The important thing is that your doctor and you are aware that PCOS may increases your risk of certain pregnancy-related conditions and that your pregnancy should be closely monitored.

When you get pregnant, probably the best thing you can do is be diligent about seeing your doctor, reporting anything that seems unusual and insisting on early and regular monitoring – especially of blood sugar and blood pressure – and to eat well, pace yourself (but still get good exercise) and do all the things that should be done by any pregnant woman. Use the five checkpoints to a positive pregnancy below as a reference to keep yourself on track.

1. CARRY ON EATING WELL

If you've been following our PCOS diet guidelines, good for you. Keep it going now that you're pregnant, as it's great for your health and the health of your baby. It might also be a good idea to ask your doctor for some pregnancy diet information and advice.

It's particularly important that you take a 400-mg folic acid supplement at least a month before becoming pregnant and three months after conception, as this reduces your baby's chances of neural tube defects such as spina bifida.

You need 1,200 to 1,300mg of calcium every day throughout your pregnancy – about a third more than usual. Milk, yoghurt and cheese are high in calcium, as are green leafy veggies, tofu and tinned fish with bones.

You also need to make sure you get enough good-quality protein, iron, fibre and Omega 3 fatty acids. You need extra iron to produce the extra blood needed by your baby. Good food sources include chicken, eggs and spinach. Constipation can be a problem during pregnancy, so eat lots of foods high in fibre. Expectant mothers should eat no more than two portions of oily fish a week, because of the pollutants they contain. They should also avoid shark, swordfish and tuna because of the high mercury levels, as well as alcohol, raw or overcooked foods, soft cheeses and liver.

2. MANAGE YOUR WEIGHT

Weighing during pregnancy has gone out with the ark, but gaining too much weight during pregnancy has been linked to miscarriage, so try to stay within the recommended range of weight gain for your height and build, and don't use pregnancy as an excuse to binge. The idea that you need to eat for two is outdated. You don't need any extra calories in the first six months, and even in the last three you only need a couple of hundred extra a day.

▷ PREGNANCY WEIGHT-GAIN GUIDELINES

If you're underweight for your weight and height (BMI < 19.8) or if you're a teenager, the recommended total weight gain would between 28 and 45 lb.

If you're normal weight your recommended total weight gain would be between 25 and 35 lb.

If you're overweight (BMI > 26) your recommended weight gain would be between 20 (15 if you're obese) and 25 lb.

If you're expecting more than one baby your weight-gain guidelines need to be discussed with your doctor, but are usually in the range of 35 to 45 lb.

Don't restrict your intake either – even if you entered your pregnancy overweight. Dieting during pregnancy is completely not on. What we are talking about is healthy eating. If you gain under 20 lb your baby is more likely to be premature and at risk of growth problems. Your baby needs a constant supply of nutrients every day, and can't get all he or she needs from your fat stores. If you gain the recommended amount of weight for your height and build, you're most likely to produce the healthiest-weight baby.

3. GET RID OF UNHEALTHY HABITS

Avoid cigarette smoking, alcohol and caffeine. You don't need anything that could compromise your pregnancy or make symptoms of PCOS worse. And ditch unhealthy junk food and foods high in sugar, salt and saturated fats. Remember, though, that a balanced diet contains a wide variety of foods, and the 80/20 rules still applies. Just because you're pregnant doesn't mean you have to become a food saint. You can enjoy the odd indulgence!

4. EXERCISE REGULARLY AND GENTLY

Don't take nine months off from your health-boosting PCOS-beating exercise routine just because you're pregnant. Obviously you need to adapt your routine to ensure it's safe and gentle, but there's no reason to be inactive. Consult your doctor for advice.

5. REDUCE STRESS

There's a wealth of evidence to suggest that a baby is aware of its mother's emotions in the womb, and that a stressful life during pregnancy can affect a baby's neurological circuitry for good. There's also evidence from a new study on stress and early miscarriage.[21] So cut down on stress in all areas of your life. Make room for your pregnancy. Don't power on regardless. Take time to relax for a minimum of 30 minutes a day. And, as you do, visualize your baby safe and secure in your womb.

Take some time for yourself, too. Your pregnancy can be an amazing opportunity to learn the importance of self-nurturing and to plant the roots of self-love so deep that when you become a mother you will be able to replenish yourself and give authentically to your child without losing yourself. Sometimes in the flurry of responsibilities we forget to take time for ourselves. Use the stress-busting suggestions in Part 3 (Chapter 15) as a starting point.

Above all, listen to your body. It will tell you when you aren't taking care of yourself. If you're tired, rest. If you're hungry, eat. If you feel stiff, have a stretch. If you're worried about anything, talk to your doctor. If you think you could have a problem, get it evaluated. In the past you may have been able to struggle on regardless when symptoms of PCOS flared up or you felt unwell, but you simply can't do that anymore because life isn't just about you anymore – it's about you and your future child.

CHAPTER 13
FINE-TUNING YOUR TAILOR-MADE PLAN

Not every woman with PCOS is the same. Eating healthily, exercising regularly, doing your lifestyle detox and working out which natural therapies work for you will certainly help keep you in optimum health now and protect you in the future. But if you have a particular symptom that's a special cause for concern, this chapter shows how your doctor and natural therapies can help you address it.

As always, only use any herbs or dietary supplements under the care of a health professional or qualified herbalist, and inform your doctor about anything you're taking, especially if you have a history of diabetes or heart disease, or are pregnant or hoping to be. For more advice about all the supplements, herbs and natural therapies mentioned in this chapter, see Chapter 9.

ACNE

Acne isn't necessarily something you grow out of. One study indicates that up to 50 per cent of adults between the ages of 20 and 40 have some form of acne. In one study, over 80 per cent of women who were referred to a dermatology clinic for acne were found to have PCOS. This isn't to say that all women with PCOS have acne – the figure is thought to be around 30 to 40 per cent.

According to Anthony Chu, senior dermatologist at the Imperial College of Science, Technology and Medicine, Hammersmith Hospital in London, the cause of acne is *not* chocolate, fatty foods, cakes or sweets (although sometimes they can make the condition worse), nor poor hygiene (which will aggravate the problem but won't cause it). The cause is thought to be an increase in the skin's oil production. This oil, called *sebum*, is made by the sebaceous glands in the skin, which react to the male hormone testosterone. Even though many women with PCOS have slightly higher levels of testosterone in their bloodstream, some women with acne have no more than usual. So it seems that women with PCOS who also have acne have sebaceous glands that are extra-sensitive to normal levels of testosterone. Once the excess oil blocks the pores, it can form blackheads and attract bacteria. Pus can then collect at the site as white blood cells rush to fight off the infection.

For women with PCOS who have acne, the usual treatment is the contraceptive pill Dianette or Yasmin for at least six months, due to the anti-androgenic effects which can help to prevent sebaceous glands being overstimulated. Most women see a beneficial effect on acne in three months. (See Chapters 4 and 5 for more information about oral contraceptives and acne.)

Spironaclactone is another medication used to treat stubborn acne, but as it can cause irregular periods it's often given alongside the contraceptive pill.

Other medications aimed at acne include flutamide and finasteride – if you take them, side-effects can include mood swings, loss of libido and fatigue. Monitor your health. Your doctor may also prescribe topical cleansers such as benzoyl peroxide or axelaic acid to clear out pores, astringents to tighten pores, oral antibiotics to decrease skin bacteria and oral agents such as Retin A, which alter the shedding of the skin cells.

Although helpful, these medications don't get to the core of the problem: hormonal imbalance. The best way to do this is with your diet and lifestyle.

DIETARY RECOMMENDATIONS

Eating the PCOS diet we've recommended is a great start for helping your skin fight off inflammation and infection and to repair scar tissue. Other acne powerfoods are:

- Sulphur-rich foods such as eggs, onion and garlic
- Carrot, cabbage, watercress, spinach and parsley juice
- Antibacterial zinc: Good food sources are shellfish, soybean and sunflower seeds, and raw nuts
- Skin-repairing EFAs: Flaxseed oil, hempseed oil and oily fish are good sources
- Antibiotic garlic
- Vitamin E can improve skin's elasticity. Dabbing vitamin E oil (from a pierced capsule) on acne and scars can help them to heal.

LIFESTYLE CHANGES

Exercise for acne is important because it encourages a healthy blood flow to your face which can help flush out toxins. It also reduces the amount of free androgens in the bloodstream – one of the triggers of PCOS acne.

NATURAL ACNE TREATMENTS

- A 5 per cent solution of tea tree oil has been found to be as effective as a 5 per cent solution of benzoyl peroxide for most cases of acne, and has no side-effects. Use a tea tree moisturizer.
- Kombucha tea has anti-bacterial and immune-boosting qualities. You can dab it on or drink it.
- Pure aloe vera gel is anti-bacterial, soothes spots and heals scars.
- Witch hazel is soothing and cooling for angry and inflamed acne
- Antibiotic echinacea – dab a cream on the affected skin daily
- Antioxidant ketsugo appears to be able to regulate the production of sebum and soften the skin
- If your acne is mild to moderate, lavender, red clover and strawberry leaves can be used in a 'steam sauna' – but not if your acne is severe.
- The homoeopathic remedy pulsatilla is for acne which is worse at puberty and before menstruation. Kali brom is for itchy spots on the face, chest and shoulders brought about by hormonal changes. If you aren't sure about a homoeopathic remedy, consult a practitioner.
- Light therapy, which involves shining different types of light on the acne, from UV to simply coloured light, can help. Red lights have been shown to open capillaries and boost circulation, while blue light has the opposite effect. Ask a dermatologist about it.

SKIN TAGS AND COLOURATION

Some women with PCOS are prone to skin tags (*acrochordon* or a *cutaneous papilloma*) which are linked to weight gain and insulin resistance; they are small tags of skin that may have a stalk and usually appear on the eyelids, neck, armpits, upper chest and groin. Skin tags are almost always benign, and removal is generally cosmetic so insurance companies usually don't pay. The tags can be removed by surgery, or frozen or sutured off, but they may grow quickly back.

One alternative is to consider herbal remedies such as bloodroot (*Sanguinaria canadensis*). The red juice from the root is poisonous when taken internally, but used externally has a unique ability to dissolve abnormal growths without disturbing normal tissue. You can buy bloodroot in powdered form or as a paste. Apply it to the growth and then cover with a bandage. Be very careful though to check with a qualified medical herbalist and your doctor before using, and follow package directions carefully.

Acanthosis nigricans (AN) is a discoloration of the skin (often dark) on the neck, under the armpits, along the waistline, around the groin, on the knuckles, elbows and toes. Some women with more severe cases may have darkened areas around the neck, nose, eyes and cheeks.

This isn't a skin infection or disease, but an indicator of possible insulin resistance, as higher-than-normal insulin levels in the bloodstream can cause it. There's no skin treatment that will get rid of AN, but overexposure to the sun can make it worse. It may lighten up and go away by treating the root cause: insulin resistance.

BLOATING

Do you feel puffed out and bloated before a period? Do you sometimes feel sluggish and heavy round your ankles, feet and waist? Many women with PCOS get fluid retention, and it can make your weight fluctuate.

Water retention isn't the same as weight gain. When you retain water you do gain weight because your body holds on to water, but in time the body will flush out the water and your weight will stabilize. On the other hand, fat can be permanent unless you make an effort to shift it.

Fluid retention can be a symptom of hormonal imbalance, especially when there's too much oestrogen circulating without the balancing effect of progesterone, which is often the case for women with PCOS and irregular periods. It can also be the result of excess sodium, which causes the body to retain excess fluid, and to poor vitamin and mineral intake. Many women suffer from fluid retention just before their periods because there's a temporary rise in the body's sodium level. Food allergies may also be a cause.

Over-the-counter diuretics aren't really a good idea as they leach valuable nutrients from your body. Try these self-help ideas:

- Cut down on salt
- Increase your water intake – this helps your body dilute the salt in your tissues and allows you to excrete more water and salt. Aim to drink 2–3 litres a day.
- Reduce your caffeine intake
- Boost your potassium levels – reach for those bananas, tomatoes, green leafy vegetables, wholegrain and fresh fruits
- Use grapeseed extract.

SUPPLEMENTS

Vitamin B$_6$, when taken as a B complex supplement, is a tried-and-tested remedy for water retention.

You can also try evening primrose oil or a tincture of *Agnus castus*. For aromatherapy, try Roman chamomile in your bath or as a massage oil.

CONSTIPATION/DIGESTIVE PROBLEMS

Many women with PCOS have digestive problems, especially constipation and IBS (irritable bowel syndrome), and this is currently being researched. It may be linked to with the slightly lowered metabolic rate after a meal, which is common among women with PCOS, and slows digestion. Food takes longer to digest, or isn't digested efficiently, and this can lead to digestive problems.

Certain drugs, such as antibiotics, can alleviate malabsorption problems, but dietary modification should be your first line of treatment. Healthy eating according to our diet guidelines, making sure you get enough fibre and drinking plenty of water are the best solutions for digestive complaints. Also watch out for food allergies and certain foods that trigger problems: Lactose (found in milk and dairy products) is a common culprit, while alcohol and tobacco can irritate the linings of the stomach and colon. When an intestinal upset occurs, make your diet blander than usual. Stick to alkaline foods such as fruits and vegetables, and avoid acid-forming foods such as meat, fish, eggs, cheese, grains, bread, flour, sugar, peas, beans, legumes, tea, coffee, alcohol and milk.

Research has also found that people who practise stress management have fewer and less severe attacks, and deep breathing exercises can help. Chewing your food well and taking time when you eat, as well as avoiding food a few hours before bedtime, can also help.

Nettle tea, slippery elm tea, rhubarb root and other herbal formulas specifically designed for constipation can be found in your local health food stores. The best herb for IBS is gentiana root. Peppermint oil capsules can be helpful, too.

Finally, food-combining might help some women with PCOS. Paying attention to the mix of alkaline- and acid-forming foods in every meal might make it easier for your body to digest food and balance your intake. Be aware, though, that the original William Hay diet is very complex and rigid – go for more modern interpretations that explains it more simply. There are some helpful books on food combining listed in the Resources chapter (page 385).

DEPRESSION

See Chapter 16.

DIABETES/INSULIN RESISTANCE

There's evidence that a diet rich in high-fibre, low-GI complex carbohydrates can lower the risk of diabetes. We've said it before but we'll say it again: the nutritional and lifestyle approach that is the focus of this book is fundamental if you have diabetes or insulin resistance. Everything you eat and drink affects your blood sugar levels and the way you feel.

Basically the diet recommended by both the British and American Diabetic Associations is simply a healthy diet. The majority of nutritional and lifestyle guidelines for people with diabetes are exactly the same as for any women looking after their present and future health. There isn't any need to buy special 'diabetic' foods.

A wholesome, nutritious diet is the best way to boost your overall health and keep insulin resistance at bay, but another part of the therapeutic answer may lie in dietary supplements. Super-charging your diet with vitamins and minerals can help you manage glucose levels, improve insulin efficiency and bring you closer to optimum health. The most important nutrients in this regard include the B vitamins, the antioxidant vitamins A, C and E, and the minerals selenium, zinc, magnesium and chromium.

Metformin treatment can be long term, but although often prescribed for women with PCOS who are insulin resistant it isn't yet a licensed treatment for PCOS in the UK and can only be prescribed by a specialist in reproductive medicine.

Supplementing with essential fatty acids (EFAs) may also be wise, as research has shown that EFAs can reduce the risk of many diseases, diabetes included.

Finally, studies on rats have shown that alpha lipoic acid can increase the efficiency of insulin. Dosages ranging from 100 to 300mg daily may be beneficial – although women with diabetes are likely to benefit from a higher dose – around 600mg daily.

NATURAL THERAPIES FOR DIABETES

Stress management is an important part of any self-help program if you have insulin resistance/diabetes. Techniques such as tai chi and meditation will help reduce adrenaline and cortisol levels – both hormones which raise blood glucose levels – and consequently improve diabetes control.

The World Health Organization endorses the use of acupuncture as a complementary treatment for diabetes. Physical therapies which can reduce or alleviate some of the painful complications of diabetes, such as those affecting the nerves or circulation, are acupuncture, acupressure, aromatherapy, herbal remedies, reflexology and yoga.[1]

A number of herbs can help stabilize glucose blood sugar levels. Two studies published in the *European Journal of Clinical Nutrition* reported that fenugreek improves glucose tolerance. Cinnamon may also be helpful, according to US researchers. Ginseng is currently under investigation as a treatment for diabetes. Research from Canada has shown that ginseng can reduce the rapid rise in blood sugar levels when taken after a meal.

Other herbs often used by medical herbalists tailor-making prescriptions for people with insulin resistance/diabetes include cedar berries, Gymnema sylvestre, bitter melon, garlic, juniper berries, cayenne pepper, huckleberry, milk thistle, bitter lemon and Pycnogenol.

Warning:
Because some herbs can have a rapid effect on blood sugar levels, and because this effect will vary from person to person, it's important to talk to your doctor before trying any herbal therapy. If you're on other medication, some herbs may interact with it – get your doctor involved.

ENDOMETRIOSIS

Endometriosis is a common and often painful disorder where cells that usually form your womb lining (endometrium) migrate outside your womb and attach themselves to other organs – most commonly your fallopian tubes, ovaries or the tissue lining your pelvis. When your usual monthly hormonal cycle triggers a period, this migrated womb-lining tissue continues to act in its normal way: it thickens, breaks down and bleeds each month as your hormone levels rise and fall. Because it can't exit through your vagina as usual, however, it becomes trapped, and can form scar tissue and even cysts that bind internal organs together and cause not only pain but also fertility problems, as scars and adhesions on ovaries or fallopian tubes can prevent pregnancy.

It's not uncommon to see both PCOS and endometriosis in the same woman, and some experts believe they must be linked. Dr Samuel Thatcher lists PCOS as one of the risk factors for endometriosis. Both are linked to hormone imbalance, typically excess amounts of oestrogen – and it's this high level of oestrogen which often makes symptoms of endometriosis worse for women who also have PCOS.

Endometriosis may improve for some women during pregnancy, when progesterone overtakes oestrogen and there are no periods. Medical treatments involve creating a state of 'pseudo pregnancy' or the menopause to limit the production of oestrogen; surgical treatments, in severe cases, can involve removal of the ovaries. Both PCOS and endometriosis respond well to self-help measures such as the healthy diet, regular exercise and stress-management advice recommended in this book, combined with the recommended care from your healthcare practitioner.

FATIGUE

Fatigue isn't recognized as a symptom of PCOS, but many women with PCOS say they feel tired and low a lot of the time. Blood sugar problems can often leave you feeling tired, and coping with the stresses of PCOS can leave you feeling low – which can sap your energy levels, too. As well as helping to stabilize blood sugar by eating according to the PCOS guidelines in Chapter 6, try these fatigue-busting ideas:

- Avoid energy-robbers that interfere with your blood sugar levels: sugar, alcohol, saturated fats, caffeine, white flour products and highly processed foods. Pesticides, hormones and additives rob food of its energy potential.
- Make sure you drink enough water throughout the day.
- The most important energy foods are those rich in B complex vitamins, found in abundance in wholegrains such as millet, buckwheat, rye and quinoa, corn, alfalfa and barley. If these grains are sprouted their energy quotient is increased many times. Sprouting is a simple process where you soak, then germinate and finally eat the growing live sprouts. Fresh, green leafy vegetables are also rich in vitamin B.
- If you drink a lot of tea, have heavy periods and are a vegetarian, you could have iron-deficiency anaemia – a lack of red blood cells to carry oxygen around your body. Your doctor can check your iron levels. To avoid iron-deficiency anaemia, replace tea with herbal drinks and eat iron-rich wholegrains and wheat germ, and lots of vitamin C-rich green leafy vegetables. Allow yourself to have a small portion of red

meat now and again, and if you're a vegetarian make sure your soya milk and cereals are iron fortified and you snack on iron-rich apricots or a small bar of dark chocolate.

- Other nutrients essential for energy production include magnesium (found in green vegetables, nuts and seeds), copper (found in oats, salmon and mushrooms), co-enzyme Q10 (found in spinach, beef and peanuts) and EFAs (found in flaxseeds and hempseeds).

- Sea vegetables or sea weed are a highly digestible source of minerals. They can improve digestion and enhance mental energy. Wild blue green algae contains virtually every nutrient known to man and can provide a feeling of well-being and vitality.

- Laugh more. Keep your sense of humour well stimulated: spend time with people who make you feel happy, watch comedies on TV or the stage, dance to upbeat music – whatever makes you smile.

- Get creative. Are you passionate about something? When you're focused and motivated you feel alert and energized. Play thinking games, read a good book, take up a new interest or hobby, learn a new language, join a debating society, enrol in an evening class – anything that can help keep your mind stimulated and fully awake.

- Lime essential oil, lemon or peppermint in your morning bath can be invigorating, and a cup of peppermint, lemon or ginger tea is a great alternative pick-me-up rather than energy-draining coffee or tea.

- There are also a number of therapies you might like to experiment with that are thought to boost energy, including yoga, tai chi, massage, aromatherapy and acupuncture.

- Get some fresh air. When you're exposed to sunlight not only do you get a top-up of energy-boosting vitamin D but your body starts to produce serotonin, which makes you feel alert and happy. Get outside whenever you can – even in winter, wrapped up warm, for a walk in the day's brightness.

FERTILITY PROBLEMS

See Chapter 12.

HAIR LOSS

Have you noticed overall thinning of your hair or thinning at the corners above the temple? Is your hair going 'see-through' – the sort of hair that appears as a fine fuzzy halo when a light shines on it? This is called *alopecia androgenetica* and is the female version of male-pattern baldness. Remember, though, it's normal to lose around a hundred hairs a day. If you think you're losing more than this, then you probably have alopecia.

According to Dr David Fenton, Consultant Dermatologist at St Thomas's Hospital, London,

'Women with PCOS can get hair loss and thinning due to excess androgens in the bloodstream. Mostly women with PCOS first notice thinning on the top of the head, but the shedding may be variable due to when ovulation occurs and when it doesn't.'

Dr Fenton believes that the contraceptive pill can cause an increased shedding of hair, though he does say that this often evens out as the body adjusts to the new hormonal balance and new hair-growth cycles begin. Balancing out hormonal cycles in PCOS through eating a healthy diet is the best way to tackle the problem, regardless of whether you take the Pill or any other anti-androgen medication on top.

DIETARY STRATEGIES FOR THINNING HAIR

Hair loss can be made worse by nutritional deficiencies, especially a lack of iron, vitamin B_1, vitamin C, vitamin E, zinc or lysine (an amino acid). Follow the diet recommendations in this book. Make sure you don't go short on EFAs or water. Dry hair that lacks shine and breaks easily is often a sign of lack of EFAs. Since hair is 98 per cent protein, make sure you're eating enough lean fish, poultry and low-fat dairy or eggs. And include in your diet foods that are rich in biotin such as brewer's yeast, brown rice, green peas, lentils, oats, soybeans, sunflower seeds and walnuts.

Avoid foods containing raw eggs, which are high in avidin, a protein that prevents biotin being absorbed. Cooked eggs are fine. The grain alfalfa, particularly in its sprouted form, has long been believed to stimulate hair growth. Eat more iron-rich foods, from lean organic meats to apricots, dark green and dark red vegetables.

Try not to eat too many cereal grains or soya products if you're losing hair, as these contain substances called phylates which can cause deficiency in minerals like calcium, iron and zinc. Stick to *no more* than one *small* portion of soya and cereal grains a day.

OTHER IDEAS

- Scalp massage (easy when you're shampooing your hair) can be helpful. Scottish researchers have found that 44 per cent of alopecia patients massaging their heads daily with a mixture of thyme, lavender, tea tree and cedarwood essential oils in a carrier oil found a big improvement in their symptoms over 7 months compared with just 15 per cent of those using carrier oils alone.

- Some natural practitioners prescribe the mineral silicon to prevent hair loss. Horsetail is a good source of silicon.

- Liquorice extract, taken orally or used topically in a cream from a Traditional Chinese Medicine (TCM) practitioner, may help prevent hair loss.

- TCM holds that the kidneys reflect the quality of your hair. Taking supplements to support your kidneys (see Chapter 9) is important.

- Use apple cider vinegar and sage tea as a rinse to help make hair shiny, or try nettle tea. For dark hair, adding a teaspoon of vinegar or rosemary can add shine. To lighten and brighten blonde hair, use chamomile.

- Regaine is a hair treatment available from your pharmacy for women with a family history of hair loss who have a general thinning of hair at the top of the scalp. If you're thinking of trying Regaine, be sure to consult with your doctor first as it isn't recommended for women with hypertension. It may also interact with certain medications and isn't advisable if you're pregnant or hoping to be. After 16–32 weeks of daily application you may begin to see positive results.

HIRSUTISM (EXCESS HAIR)

The healthy diet guidelines in this book will help balance your hormones and reduce the androgen imbalance that triggers hirsutism. Studies show that with a healthy diet and weight loss, symptoms of PCOS such as hirsutism decrease. Exercise can also improve hirsutism because the fitter you become the lower your body fat and the better your insulin and glucose control. This in turn reduces the amount of testosterone that your ovary produces and that is circulating in your bloodstream.

If you're spending too much time plucking, waxing and shaving, in addition to your basic healthy diet your doctor could help by prescribing the contraceptive pill. (For more information on what your doctor can offer if you have hirsutism, see Chapter 5.)

A medical herbalist can also help, often by prescribing saw palmetto – usually in combination with other herbs in a tailor-made prescription.

HYPERTENSION

If you've got PCOS, research suggests your risk of hypertension (high blood pressure) is higher than normal. This is because many of the symptoms associated with PCOS – weight gain, high cholesterol and insulin resistance – are known to be risk factors for cardiovascular disease and its precursor, high blood pressure.

The treatment and prevention of high blood pressure, or hypertension, begins with the diet and lifestyle changes recommended in this book: stop smoking, eat a healthy diet, lose weight if you've weight to lose, and exercise more. Your doctor normally won't consider medication until at least a six-month trial of healthy diet and regular exercise has been attempted. It's especially important to eat more antioxidants such as vitamins C, E, A, B, zinc and selenium, as these all help protect against free radical damage to the arteries, a major cause of high blood pressure.

If you need drug therapy there are a variety of anti-hypertensive drugs available; unfortunately, none of them is perfect. Most studies have been done on men and older women; more studies need to be done on women under the age of 50. You may find that you have to try several different drugs to find the one that best suits you.

Diuretics work by flushing sodium and water from your body, and if you've got PCOS spironolactone may be the best option. Beta blockers widen blood vessels and ease the heart's pumping action, but they may not be the best choice as they make glucose intolerance worse. Angiotensin converting enzyme (ACE) inhibitors (e.g. Lotensin, Accupril, Monopril, Zestril and Captopril) reduce the production of angiotensin, a chemical that causes the arteries to constrict. The side-effects range from a dry throat and/or cough to skin rash. They are the drug of choice for women with insulin resistance/diabetes, and therefore probably the best drug option if you've got PCOS.

Generally, once you start blood pressure medication you need to stay on it for the rest of your life, even after your blood pressure returns to normal. If you were to stop treatment, your reading would probably climb right back to an unhealthy level. The good news is that you may be able to reduce your dosage – once your blood pressure stays in the normal range (120/80) for at least a year.

NON-PRESCRIPTION SUPPLEMENTS

Certain herbs and supplements may lower blood pressure as effectively as prescription pharmaceuticals, especially in combination with the lifestyle strategies we recommend in this book. Even better, natural remedies tend to have fewer side-effects than drugs. On the other hand, they do work more slowly than conventional medications and they can sometimes cause troublesome interactions with other drugs. For these reasons always consult a doctor who is knowledgeable about herbs and nutritional supplements before adding them to your self-care regime.

- Garlic – Take four to six 600-mg garlic capsules or tablets every day can help
- Co-enzyme Q10 – 100g a day taken with meals
- Fish oil – thought to thin the blood
- Chromium – there's a demonstrable lack of chromium in people who die of heart disease. If you have high blood pressure, 400–800mcg chromium picolinate daily may be beneficial.
- Calcium – you know it helps protect against osteoporosis, but is also helps rein in blood pressure
- Potassium – discourages LDL ('bad') cholesterol from sticking to artery walls – eat a small banana a day.
- Ginkgo – Dilates the peripheral blood vessels and thins the blood
- Hawthorn – look for capsules that are standardized as a flavonoid called vitexin, and follow instructions for usage. Do not use for more than four weeks without having a medical check-up.

- Finally, celery deserves a special mention as it may contain substances (3-n-butyl phthalide) that can help lower blood pressure. Add celery to salads, soups and meat or fish dishes, or eat with vegetable dips.

IRREGULAR PERIODS

In addition to PCOS, poor eating habits (resulting in vitamin and mineral deficiencies), wild swings in weight, eating a lot of processed carbohydrates and very low-fat diets can all affect your periods, as can stress. If you have PCOS and don't ovulate for several months, your ovaries' secretion of oestrogen becomes erratic and you may have surges of the hormone which cause irregular, heavy and painful bleeds. If you don't want to go on the Pill, either because it doesn't agree with you or you want to regularize your periods in order to get pregnant, natural progesterone cream can help regulate your cycle. The progesterone from skin cream is absorbed into your bloodstream. If you're having no periods at all you need to apply the cream daily for several months to feel an effect. If you have irregular periods you need to use the cream for three weeks out of every four. If your periods are very heavy confine the cream to the second half of your menstrual cycle. You can get progesterone cream on prescription from your doctor in the UK; in the US it's readily available (see Resources, page 385). It's important to work with your doctor if you want to use natural progesterone cream. It's called 'natural' but it's still a drug, and until studies prove otherwise its use remains controversial. Too much of any hormone can have the opposite effect from the one desired.

There are also things you can do to help yourself:

- First and foremost, eat a healthy diet according to the guidelines in this book

- Take a multivitamin and -mineral that includes B vitamins, zinc, vitamin C, beta carotene and vitamin E.

- You might also want to take an additional vitamin B_6 and zinc supplement, as studies have deficiencies to irregular periods. Also, EFAs have been proven to help regulate the cycle: nutritionist Marilyn Glenville advises supplementing with 150mg of Omega 6 and at least 2g of Omega 3 a day.

- Maintain a healthy body weight (see Chapter 11).

- Massage your abdomen with lavender or melissa oil if periods are irregular, rose or cypress oil if periods are heavy, marjoram oil or a warm compress placed on your abdomen if your periods are painful. Use a total of 2 drops of essential oil in a teaspoon of carrier oil for massage, up to 4 drops for a bath.

- Try a warm bath with a couple of drops of geranium (mood-lifting) chamomile (pain-killing) and clary sage (muscle-relaxant) oils to ease cramping and soothe pain. You could also try the good old hot water bottle. Willow bark and kava kava tablets are natural alternatives to aspirin and are available from health food stores and herbalists.

- Graphites or actaea racemosa are often prescribed for irregular periods, but there are so many causes of irregular periods that remedies should be prescribed only by a homoeopath on an individual basis. The exception is a missed period resulting from sudden emotional shock, when you can try aconite 30c twice a day for two to three days. If there's no relief after a week, see a practitioner.

- If your periods have stopped completely or your ovulation pattern is irregular, the herb *Agnus castus* can be helpful. Other useful herbs that a medical herbalist might prescribe include false unicorn root, blue cohosh, wild yam, dong quai, dandelion, licorice, motherwort, siberian ginseng and squaw vine. You might even be prescribed raspberry leaf tea to improve circulation.

- Studies have shown that acupuncture can be very effective at relieving pain and regulating the hormonal system. Yoga can also restore hormonal balance, and there are specific exercises to ease tension in the lower abdomen. Deep breathing and stretching can help relax your muscles and your mind and increase the blood flow to the pelvic region.

THYROID PROBLEMS

Many of the symptoms and risk factors for thyroid disorders mirror those of PCOS, and since all the hormonal systems in our body are interconnected it's possible that our risk is potentially higher than a woman without PCOS. In fact, because the conditions are so similar your doctor may want to rule out thyroid disorder before a diagnosis of PCOS can be made.

Some experts believe that women with PCOS have a dysfunction of the insulin system and thyroid along with dysfunctional ovaries. An interesting study[2] from the Universita degli Studi di Roma in Italy investigated the relationship between polycystic ovary syndrome, hypothyroidism and insulin-resistance and revealed how, by submitting patients to a specific therapy for any one of the three conditions, the researchers could obtain an improvement in the others.

If you're feeling tired for no reason and suffer from headaches, low libido, mood swings, dry skin, hair loss, weight gain, high cholesterol, poor concentration and intolerance to cold, you may be suffering from hypothyroidism or reduced thyroid function. Basically your thyroid gland isn't producing the right amount of hormones, and this is upsetting the delicate biochemical balance in your body.

Standard treatment for an underactive thyroid involves daily use of the synthetic drug levothyroxine. This oral medication can restore adequate hormone levels and shift your body back into balance. Although most doctors recommend synthetic extracts, natural extracts such as Westhroid and Armour hormone, containing thyroid glands from animals, are also available.

OTHER RECOMMENDATIONS

- Naturopathic Consultant Martin Budd recommends a low-fat and low-sugar diet that uses the glycaemic index to make food choices. A diet very similar, in fact, to that followed in the eastern Mediterranean, where the incidence of diabetes and hypothyroidism is low. The term 'Mediterranean Triad' was first coined by Paul Kendrick to describe the three key elements of the regional diets of Greece, Italy and southern France: wholegrain products, fresh fruits and vegetables, and less total fat and sugar (by substituting olive oil and other oils for solid fats and replacing red meat with lean meat). Sound familiar?
- Avoid fluoride (including that found in toothpaste and tap water) and chlorine (also found in tap water). Chlorine and fluoride are chemically related and can block receptors in the thyroid gland, resulting in reduced thyroid function.
- Supplements include kelp, made from seaweed, because it contains iodine (the basic substance of thyroid hormones), vitamin B complex,

brewer's yeast (rich in B vitamins and EFAs), vitamins A, C and E and the minerals selenium, manganese, copper, iron and zinc

- A medical herbalist might recommend the herbs bayberry, black cohosh and golden seal in a tailor-made prescription.

NATURAL THERAPIES FOR THYROID

As with PCOS, all thyroid symptoms have an impact on your mind as well as your body, with depression a common symptom. Therapies that act on your body via your mind and vice versa are therefore likely to be particularly helpful. Yoga and tai chi are sometimes known as 'moving meditation' and may help to raise energy levels and mood. Aromatherapy is mood-restorative too. Rosemary, for example, can relax away tension, basil lifts your mood, lavender is relaxing and lemon balm can help you sleep peacefully.

One of the few alternative therapies that has been studied scientifically in relation to thyroid problems is autogenic training (see page 174). This therapy is particularly useful for mild anxiety states. The techniques have been found to lower heart rate and blood pressure and improve emotional balance. As far as specific thyroid symptoms are concerned, research has shown that a number of typical symptoms of an overactive thyroid diminish over the course of autogenic training treatment.

WEIGHT GAIN

See Chapter 11.

PART THREE
TAKING CHARGE OF PCOS: NURTURING YOUR EMOTIONS AND SPIRIT

CHAPTER 14
PREPARING TO TAKE CONTROL

The emotional distress that accompanies PCOS symptoms should never be underestimated. But how can you find ways to turn your negative feelings about PCOS into motivation to change and help yourself get well? That's what this chapter is all about.

GETTING MOTIVATED FOR CHANGE

Working to keep symptoms and the long-term health risks of PCOS at bay is a project for life. It won't always be easy and there will be times when you feel like giving up, so how can you get – and stay – motivated?

The motivation to change your lifestyle has to come from inside you. To get the job done it's important that you change your diet and lifestyle because you *want* to and not because your doctor has advised it or your loved ones urge it. Where does this conviction come from?

1. A desire to improve and maintain your health and specifically to control your symptoms, prevent the possibility of diabetes and heart disease and maximize your chances of health and a long life.
2. A desire to lose weight, if you have weight to lose, and look your physical best.
3. A desire to feel good mentally – to be more confident, have more self-esteem and experience all-round feelings of accomplishment, fulfilment and satisfaction.

Three excellent reasons, and three powerful motivators: better health, improved body image, and an increased sense of mental and emotional well-being.

You can help yourself get through the bad days and celebrate good days by gathering together your own support network. This can come ready-made in the form of a self-help group, or it can be a web of people you talk to about PCOS. Besides partners, family, friends and healthcare workers, an excellent place to turn for support is other women with PCOS. Verity and PCOSupport, as well as e-groups on the internet, certainly offer this type of help and support.

FIND YOUR TRIGGER

Most of us are afraid of change and keep putting it off. There needs to be more pain than pleasure before we make the effort – like the smoker who only gives up after a heart scare, even though they've known for years that smoking is a killer.

Many women with PCOS are triggered, or warned, by something that isn't pleasant to feel or know. Did your doctor (or this book) warn you of the increased risks of PCOS? Did you realize that your insulin resistance was edging you slowly towards full-blown diabetes? Did a recent photo of yourself make you feel sad? Did you cry in the changing room while trying on new clothes? Instead of trying to downplay or ignore these triggers because of the discomfort and pain they cause, or put off your good intentions, you should relive or exaggerate these triggers so that they become a powerful driving force to propel you towards change.

GIVE UP NEGATIVE SELF-BELIEF

Another great way to keep your motivation high is positive 'self-talk'.

Personal trainers Pete Cohen and Judith Verity specialize in the power of the mind when it comes to weight loss. Here are their favourite tips for women with PCOS.

I. I'M STARTING!

Old habits really do die hard, and change of any kind is always stressful. A good way to get started on any major life change is by using 'away from' motivation.

Conjure up powerful images of how you will look and feel if things don't change in your life. Lighten Up uses the 'Scrooge' technique, where what your life could become is an incentive for change. Perhaps poor health and weight gain limit your movements? Do you feel constantly tired and low?

This helps you focus on the real reason why you want to change your eating habits. Think about how improved health and weight loss, if you need it, will improve your relationships and your self-esteem, now and in the years to come.

2. I'M SLIPPING!

In order to keep going once you've made a start you need 'towards' motivation. This time, instead of dwelling on what will happen if you don't change your eating habits, put some energy into picturing yourself in the future. Your hair is shiny, your skin soft and smooth, and your periods are regular. You feel slimmer, healthier, fitter, fully in control of your life and able to cope with anything.

But what do you do if you understand all the benefits of healthy eating you still find it hard to stay focused and committed? On page 258 you'll find some techniques and strategies you can use to help you accomplish your goals.

You then can link this vision with healthy eating or exercise sessions. See yourself eating healthy food and enjoying it. See yourself having lots of energy to exercise. This isn't something you do once. You need to do it over and over again until it becomes a habitual way of thinking on a daily basis.

3. IT TAKES SUCH A LONG TIME!

You can help yourself stay patient and positive with daily motivational statements, night and morning, such as:

'I can manage my PCOS.'

'I'm slimmer, fitter and healthier.'

'I'm looking and feeling good.'

'The quality of my life is improving every day.'

Affirmations like this won't make you slimmer or healthier, but they can help you on your way to health and happiness on a daily basis. They give you that 'oomph' factor you need to keep going.

If you're tempted to go back to old habits, like daily chocolate fixes or junk food, ask yourself what benefits you were getting from your old eating patterns, and find different ways to get them. If chocolate makes you feel comforted, give someone a hug instead. If crisps stop you feeling bored, call a friend or pick up a good book. Experiment with new ways of getting pleasure, comfort and satisfaction in your life, to carry you through until your new habits become second nature and your feelings of frustration are forgotten.

4. I'M EXCITED BUT DON'T WANT TO SET UNREALISTIC GOALS!

Congratulate yourself on a daily basis when you get something right: when you make a healthy eating choice, walk to work, whatever it is – get into the habit of patting yourself on the back. This will help you appreciate the changes you've already made without making you feel you've got to move faster than your body can cope with.

It's important to take time to listen to what your body's saying. You can do this with a diary. At the end of each week ask yourself these three questions:

1. Do I feel good?
2. Do I have lots of energy?
3. Am I enjoying my food and my exercise routine?

If the answer to any of them is 'No' it's probably time to change your routine and work towards more achievable goals.

5. I FEEL GREAT AND I WANT TO STAY THAT WAY

When you have a really good feeling about yourself and the changes you're making, acknowledge that feeling and dwell on it. If you have two regular periods in a row, for instance, or you just feel fitter and slimmer, make sure you make a mental note. We all have a tendency to dwell on the bad feelings and even seek them out. When you're feeling good or pleased with your progress, give yourself another of those pats on the back, or even treat yourself to a walk in your favourite park, a favourite movie, a day off with your partner, a phone call to a treasured friend – and remember that feeling. Spend some time daydreaming and make a mental movie of yourself looking and living a healthy life. Watch that movie over and over again.

▷ PRACTICAL TIPS FOR STAYING MOTIVATED

Here are some tips from Alex Cross and Rachel Green, counselling psychotherapists who run an emotional support group for women with PCOS (see Resources, page 385) at St Ann's Hospital, London:

'The two main ways in which our own participants managed to maintain their motivation for change was by:

1. Looking at the diet and exercise plan as an ongoing, permanent lifestyle change. If you accept that you have a condition that needs your care and attention, you stop thinking about trying to force down brown rice for six months (with one eye on the date you can stop!). You can, very slowly, think about what kind of permanent change you feel able to make. This means working out a diet and exercise plan that's best suited to who you are, and the kind of lifestyle you enjoy. Accepting that you have a health condition can also liberate you from feeling like a "fat" woman. You simply have a health condition that requires you to live a certain way.

2. It's also important to feel the lifestyle changes are to be enjoyed! Motivation remains low when you see goals as unpleasant. How can you find new pleasures in diet and exercise changes? For example, walking to work on sunny days as opposed to forcing yourself to go to the gym. Or really simple things like reducing sugar in tea over time rather than trying to go "cold turkey". Keeping goals small also helps. Even if it just means becoming aware for a period of time of the kinds of foods that you eat, and/or the kinds of temptations that are likely to fall into your path.

'Our participants also told us that knowledge of the role of insulin in diet and exercise made a huge difference to their motivation. Perhaps their ideas could help you. Many of them developed simple "rules" that they used as motivational tools. For example, "exercise reduces insulin" or "sugar increases insulin". Many found the motivation to exercise for the first time, as they finally understood that exercise wasn't just to "get the fat off", it actually lowers their insulin (and hopefully their testosterone). Exercise can therefore help to keep the hair at bay as well as help to kick-start ovulation and protect them from diabetes.

'One other tip for increasing motivation was to look at whose support they'd enlisted in the past to make changes. Can you get your friends and family to help you stay motivated?

'You need to ground the idea of "change" in realistic terms, noting that we all fluctuate between readiness and contemplation. Once you have been given permission to lapse, it's easier to avoid falling into a complete relapse. It's also then easier to start again. See your lapses as a completely natural part of the process and you'll be less tempted to give it all up.

'Finally, here are some success stories from women who have attended our group and found the motivation they needed to make lasting changes. There's nothing like hearing other women with PCOS feeling positive to give you a lift.

'"I now feel able and ready to control my symptoms through exercise and thinking about what I eat."

'"It was nice to know that there were more people like me. And I have had answers to questions that have never been answered before."

'"Talking to other women with PCOS gave me confidence and made me laugh and see good in my illness."

'"I feel more confident within myself, I am happier and not so conscious of others around me. And I have already lost weight!"

"'Before I attended the group, I didn't have a lot of knowledge about PCOS. After attending the group, I have felt more equipped to combat the symptoms of the condition."

"'It was comforting to know that there are things I can do to help make this a condition I can live with."

"'Giving us support for how we feel about living with PCOS has given us the confidence to deal with it ourselves.'"

GET SUPPORT

Perhaps the best motivator of all is to enlist the support of a healthcare team, your partner, if you have one, and your family, colleagues and friends.

You will be more successful if the changes you want to make can be adopted by everyone. If you live in a family setting you might even be able to persuade your partner, children or parents that it's a good idea that you all do it together. Once they start to notice you feeling and looking better, the chances are they will want to reap the benefits too.

'My kids will say we need brown rice and brown bread when we're in the supermarket. They say it's to keep mummy happy.'
Jodie, 36

BE GENTLE ON YOURSELF

The very fact that you're reading this book shows that you're motivated for change, but as you make changes realize that you will inevitably experience times when, no matter how hard you try, you can't lose weight or you slip back into old habits. When this happens, don't lose heart. It's all part of the healthy change process. Be gentle on yourself and don't beat yourself up; guilt and self-chastisement are pointless and demoralizing. Just tell yourself that tomorrow is another day. Then try again and get back on track.

'If I fall off the healthy eating wagon, and catch myself being angry with myself, I stop, take a deep breath, and try to imagine what I would say if I was talking to a friend who came to me in this same situation. Suddenly the way I think changes – I think, ok, now this has happened, don't let it ruin everything you've already achieved. Use it to spur yourself on to do even better from now on.'

Shauneese, 31

CHAPTER 15
STRESS AND PCOS – HOW TO LET GO AND LIVE BETTER

If you find that your PCOS symptoms get worse when you're stressed or feeling anxious, you're not alone.

Stress triggers a set of biological responses – a release of stress hormones from your adrenal gland (adrenaline and cortisol), an increase in blood sugar, flexing of the muscles, shallow breathing, rising blood pressure and rapid heart rate. All these responses are designed to help you meet physical challenges that threaten your survival, but the trouble is most modern-day stresses – missing a train or getting stuck in traffic – can't be resolved by action. You just sit there and seethe, and all the while your stress responses are on full alert.

New research supports the theory that chronic stress at work is a major risk factor in the development of heart disease and diabetes. A study published by the *British Medical Journal* (BMJ) states that it 'provides new evidence for the biological plausibility of the link between work stress and heart disease'.

Over time your adrenal glands become increasingly overworked and have difficulty producing hormones in the right amount. Too much cortisol and adrenaline triggers the release of too much testosterone, and this can drive your body towards insulin resistance, weight gain and irregular periods. Prolonged stress also affects your digestion, so you aren't getting the nutrients you need, and your immune system, so you're more likely to get colds and flu. Most importantly, your risk of heart disease increases.

Too much stress can have a negative impact on anyone's health, increasing the risk of depression, insulin resistance, diabetes, infertility, heart disease and even cancer, but if you've got PCOS you may be at even greater risk. Cortisol, the active form of the hormone, can be turned into cortisone, the inactive form, by enzymes in the body – but researchers[1] have found some women with PCOS don't have these enzymes. This means their bodies cannot process cortisol properly, which causes higher levels of testosterone to be produced. So it seems that we may not be able to deal with stress as effectively as women who don't have PCOS.

WHAT STRESS MEANS FOR YOU

PSYCHOLOGICAL EFFECTS

A continual state of stress depresses serotonin, which increases anxiety and appetite, and is a trigger for depression. Stress also diminishes your quality of life by robbing you of your sense of pleasure, self-worth, security, accomplishment and empowerment.

WEIGHT GAIN

Stress-induced cortisol, insulin resistance and numerous other factors predispose you to gain weight, especially around the middle. Abdominal fat is a predictor of diabetes and cardiovascular problems. Women with central obesity (belly fat), whether obese or not, produce more of the stress hormone cortisol than women without belly fat.[2]

High cortisol reactivity in response to stress may also lead to overeating after stress. One study[3] showed that women with a high level of cortisol reactivity consumed more calories on stressful days than those without high cortisol levels. They also ate significantly more sweet foods (refined carbohydrates).

SEXUAL FUNCTION

Stress tends to diminish sexual desire and responsiveness.

FERTILITY AND REPRODUCTIVE HORMONES

Some women who don't menstruate have higher cortisol levels than menstruating women, and cortisol also interferes with progesterone levels. Increased cortisol from stress may also disturb the timing of reproductive hormones during the menstrual cycle.[4]

EFFECTS ON PREGNANCY[5]

Stress during pregnancy has been linked to a higher risk for miscarriage, premature births and lower birthweight babies. High stress in expectant mothers can influence the baby's brain and nervous system. Stress has a constricting effect on arteries which can interfere with normal blood flow to the placenta. Stress also produces an inflammatory state that appears to reduce success with in-vitro fertilization (IVF).

More research needs to be done, but simply knowing that your stress threshold may not be high and that stress makes your symptoms worse can encourage you to take steps to stress-proof your life. Stress management is without doubt a crucial component of your plan to control PCOS and boost your health.[6]

MANAGE YOUR STRESS

Any therapy that eases mental tension, and by so doing lowers stress levels, is a plus for women with PCOS, especially those who have insulin resistance. Listed below are specific natural therapies that have been shown to help ease stress and mental tension.

Note:

To maximize your chances of success with natural therapies it's important to find a qualified practitioner who can guide and assist you. You'll find information on how to find practitioners in our Resources chapter. Some therapies, such as counselling and homoeopathy, are available on the NHS, so be sure to ask your doctor for information and advice.

DEEP BREATHING

The two exercises described here can help you change your breathing pattern from a shallow, stressed one into a pattern that promotes deep relaxation. Just three minutes of practising abdominal breathing or the calming breath exercise will usually induce a deep state of relaxation that eases away stress.

ABDOMINAL BREATHING EXERCISE

1. Place one hand on your abdomen right beneath your rib cage.
2. Inhale slowly and deeply through your nose into the 'bottom' of your lungs – in other words, send the air as low down as you can. If you're breathing from your abdomen, your hand should actually rise. Your chest should move only slightly while your abdomen expands. (In abdominal breathing, the diaphragm – the muscle that separates the lung cavity from the abdominal cavity – moves downwards. In so doing it causes the muscles surrounding the abdominal cavity to push outwards.)
3. When you've taken in a full breath, pause for a moment and then exhale slowly through your nose or mouth. Be sure to exhale fully. As you exhale, allow your whole body to just let go.

Do 10 slow, full abdominal breaths. Try to keep your breathing smooth and regular, without gulping in a big breath or letting your breath out all at once. It will help to slow down your breathing if you count to four on the inhale (1-2-3-4) and then slowly count to four again on the exhale. Remember to pause briefly at the end of each inhalation.

CALMING BREATH EXERCISE

The calming breath exercise was adapted from the ancient discipline of yoga. It's a very efficient technique for achieving a deep state of relaxation quickly.

1. Breathing from your abdomen, inhale through your nose slowly to a count of five (count slowly '1...2...3...4...5' as you inhale).
2. Pause and hold your breath to a count of five.
3. Exhale slowly, through your nose or mouth, to a count of five (or more if it takes you longer). Be sure to exhale fully.

When you've exhaled completely, take two breaths in your normal rhythm, and then repeat steps 1 through 3 in the cycle above.

Keep up the exercise for at least 3 to 5 minutes. This should involve going through at least 10 cycles of in-five, hold-five, out-five. As you continue the exercise you may notice that you can count higher when you exhale than when you inhale. Allow these variations in your counting to occur, and just continue with the exercise for up to 5 minutes. Remember to take two normal breaths between each cycle. If you start to feel light-headed, stop for 30 seconds and then start again.

Throughout the exercise, keep your breathing smooth and regular, without gulping in breaths or breathing out suddenly.

Practise the abdominal breathing or calming breath exercise for 5 minutes every day for at least two weeks. If possible, find a regular time each day to do this so that your breathing exercise becomes a habit. With practice you can learn in a short period of time to 'damp down' the physiological reactions underlying anxiety and panic.

Once you feel you've gained some mastery in the use of either technique, apply it whenever you feel stressed, anxious, or are experiencing the onset of panic symptoms. The more you can shift the centre of your breathing from your chest to your abdomen, the more consistently you will feel relaxed on an ongoing basis.

RELAXATION EXERCISES

Relaxation is a forgotten skill in today's busy world. Learn at least one relaxation exercise and you can trigger your body's relaxation response – the opposite to the stress response.

Here's one of the easiest:

1. Find a comfortable place, away from all distractions and noise. Put on some soothing, relaxing music if you like.
2. Lie down on your back or sit with your back straight.
3. Concentrate on your breathing. Make it slow and steady.
4. Inhale through your nose. Exhale through either your nose or mouth.
5. Breathe deeply, filling up the area between your navel and your rib cage. Don't breathe with your chest. Don't hold your breath.
6. Continue this breathing pattern for 5 to 10 minutes. Notice the feeling of calm throughout your whole body.
7. As you continue to breathe slowly and deeply, relax by doing the following for another 5 to 10 minutes:
8. Tighten and relax each muscle in your body. You can begin at your toes and work your way up to your head.
9. Imagine your muscle groups relaxing and becoming heavy.
10. Empty your mind of all thoughts.
11. Allow yourself to relax more and more deeply.
12. Become aware of the state of calm that surrounds you.
13. After a time, bring yourself back to alertness by moving your fingers and toes, then your hands and feet, stretching and moving your entire body. Sometimes people fall asleep during this relaxation exercise, but they usually wake up shortly afterwards.

14. Always give yourself time to return to full alertness before you drive a car or do other activities that require you to be fully alert.

VISUALIZATION

Whenever you notice yourself getting stressed, for example if you're stuck in a traffic jam, at the end of a long supermarket queue or faced with a cashpoint machine that isn't working, try to think about how important this situation really is in the scheme of things. Put it into perspective. You could also try some visualization exercises when life gets too busy and you feel everyone is making demands on you.

1. Find a quiet, private place, sit down and relax.
2. Close your eyes and become aware of your breathing.
3. When your mind and body are feeling deeply relaxed, create in your imagination a beautiful scene. Choose an outdoor setting by the beach, in the mountains, in a garden – wherever you like. Fill the scene with colour and detail and create your own wonderful holiday snaps. Let the details of the place sink in, see the sights, smell the fragrances, hear the sounds. When you have created your own little paradise, slowly return to the room and open your eyes.

Now you can go on holiday any time you like. There's no packing, no queuing, and it's free!

MEDITATION

Meditation is a good way to deal with mental and physical stress. Scientists led by Vernon Barnes at the Medical College of Georgia studied transcendental meditation with 32 healthy adults and concluded that it can lower blood pressure. Other research suggests that it can also help prevent heart disease and cancer. According to experts,[7] meditation can also ease anxiety and stress – perhaps because it shuts off your mind and allows your body to relax.

Try to make meditation a regular part of your daily routine. Set aside 10 to 20 minutes each day at the same time, if possible.

1. Choose a quiet spot where you won't be disturbed by other people or by the telephone.
2. Sit quietly in a comfortable position. Close your eyes.
3. Pick a focus word or short phrase that's firmly rooted in your personal belief system. A non-religious person might choose a neutral word like 'one', 'peace' or 'love'. Others might use the opening words of a favourite prayer such as 'Hail Mary full of Grace', 'I surrender all to you', 'Hallelujah', 'Om', etc.
4. Relax your muscles sequentially from feet to head, as in the exercise on page 269. Breathe slowly and naturally, repeating your focus word or phrase silently with each exhalation.
5. Don't worry about how well you're doing. When other thoughts come to mind, simply say, 'Oh, well,' and gently return to the repetition.
6. Continue for 10 to 20 minutes. You may open your eyes to check the time, but don't use an alarm. After you've finished, sit quietly for a

minute or so, at first with your eyes closed and then with them open. Don't stand up for a minute or two.

THE PRACTICE OF WALKING MEDITATION

If you're one of those people who finds it hard to sit or lie down for meditation, why not try the 'walking meditation' exercise? According to Jon Kabat-Zinn, Director of the Stress Reduction Clinic at the University of Massachusetts Medical Center, one simple way to bring awareness into your life is through Walking Meditation. 'This brings your attention to the actual experience of walking as you're doing it, focusing on the sensations in your feet and legs, feeling your whole body moving,' Dr Kabat-Zinn explains. 'You can also integrate awareness of your breathing with the experience.'

To do this exercise, focus your attention on each foot as it makes contact with the ground. When your mind wanders away from your feet or legs, or the feeling of your body walking, refocus your attention. To deepen your concentration, don't look around, but keep your gaze focused straight in front of you.

MASSAGE

Research[8] has shown that massage can help lower blood pressure, improve breathing, boost mood and well-being and aid circulation. Some experts believe that massage helps the brain produce endorphins, the chemicals that act as natural pain-killers. The sense of well-being you get from a massage can lower the amount of stress hormones circulating in your body.

For physical relief massage can help with chronic muscular tension and poor circulation. For mental relief massage can be thought of as a one-hour vacation from stress, a get-away from life and its challenges. During a massage you create a peaceful space and give yourself permission to relax.

As you well know, life with PCOS can be stressful, so why not book a massage every now and again and give your body a treat? Or better still, get your partner to give you a back rub at home. We highly recommend it.

YOGA

Studies suggest that yoga can help prevent hypertension and poor health. MIND, the UK's leading mental health charity, recommends yoga as the single most effective stress-buster there is.[9]

COGNITIVE BEHAVIOURAL THERAPY

CBT is a clinically proven breakthrough in mental health care. Several studies by research psychologists and psychiatrists make it clear that CBT can be effective for conditions such as stress, anxiety, depression and mood swings.

CBT combines two very effective kinds of psychotherapy – cognitive therapy and behaviour therapy. Behaviour therapy helps you weaken the connections between troublesome situations and your habitual reactions to them. It also teaches you how to calm your mind and body, so you can feel better, think more clearly and make better decisions.

Cognitive therapy teaches you how certain thinking patterns are causing your symptoms – by giving you a distorted picture of what's going on in your life and making you feel anxious, depressed or angry for no good reason, or provoking you into ill-chosen actions.

CBT provides you with very powerful tools for stopping negative thoughts and habits and getting your life on a more satisfying track.

Preliminary research suggests that CBT may be effective for women who aren't ovulating due to metabolic imbalances. A study[10] done in 2003 concluded that CBT may be most helpful for women who have high levels of stress in their lives and characteristic traits such as perfectionism, a need for social approval, and altered attitudes toward eating. The researchers sought to determine whether CBT targeted at these problems and attitudes could help restore ovarian function.

In the study CBT had the desired effect for most of the eight women treated: six resumed menstruating, one had partial recovery of ovarian function, and one had no return of ovarian function. Of the eight women in the observation (control) group, one recovered ovarian function, one had a partial recovery and six didn't recover. The members of the observation group were offered CBT after the conclusion of the study.

Research[11] is preliminary, but increasingly both scientists and mind–body experts alike believe that grumpy, pessimistic, angry people are more likely to get heart disease and suffer from poor health than people who are more relaxed and upbeat. It's important to take care of your body to beat your symptoms, but don't neglect the importance of your thoughts, emotions and state of mind. Choose to think uplifting thoughts instead of discouraging ones – remember, you get to decide what you think!

SLEEP – THE HEALING STRESSBUSTER

Stress can interfere with your sleep – but sleep is essential for your physical and emotional health. If you're well rested both mentally and physically you can cope better with the stresses of daily life. During deep sleep your body stores protein, restores energy levels and is flooded with a surge of growth hormones that are important for cell renewal and repair and good general health. Dreaming is a way for your mind to sort through problems in your daily life. Even missing just a few hours of sleep a night on a regular basis can have a detrimental effect. Life will feel more stressful and you'll be less productive. You may have problems concentrating as well as feelings of irritability and, of course, fatigue – not great if you're already feeling sluggish because of PCOS. Research has also shown that the number of natural killer cells (responsible for fighting off bacteria and viruses) are also decreased if you don't get a good night's sleep.

Sleep is even more essential for women with PCOS, because research findings[12] show that not only does sleep deprivation disrupt hormonal balance, it interferes with your blood sugar levels and increases the risk of insulin resistance and diabetes, high blood pressure, obesity, hypertension and heart disease, and may even be linked to breast cancer.[13] If all that weren't enough, research[14] also indicates that women with PCOS may be prone to sleep problems due to the hormonal fluctuations associated with the condition.

So what is good-quality sleep? Research suggests that both those who sleep for fewer than 6 hours and those who sleep for more than 7 hours become irritable. Seven hours seems to be the most beneficial, but six hours of good-quality sleep is far better than a restless 8.

AREYOU GETTING ENOUGH?

Every one has different sleep needs, but if one or more of the items on the list below applies to you, you're not getting enough good-quality sleep:

- you yawn a lot
- you fall asleep during the day
- you lack energy

- you feel drained or tired
- you need caffeine and stimulants to get you through the day
- you get dark circles under your eyes
- you find waking up difficult
- you find it hard to concentrate
- you get irritable for no reason.

The two best things you can do to improve your chances of a good night's sleep are:

STEP ONE: BOOST YOUR SEROTONIN/MELATONIN

Serotonin is manufactured within your body from the amino acid tryptophan and is found in many foods, notably eggs, cheese, milk, lean meat, fish, soybeans and potatoes. That's why the old advice to drink a glass of warm milk before you sleep can indeed work. If you prefer you can take tryptophan in supplement form (available from health food stores). You might also want to consider adding a couple of crackers or a slice of bread to your bedtime snack to help you sleep well. This is because complex carbohydrates such as rice, oats and wheat encourage insulin to be released, and when insulin is released tryptophan is, too.

In order for tryptophan to convert to serotonin/melatonin it needs vitamin B_6 so you need to ensure that you have enough vitamin B_6 in your diet. You can get B_6 from foods such as spinach, fish, lentils, avocados, carrots and potatoes. Increase your vitamin B_6 supplements during the premenstrual period, especially if you find you feel depressed at this time.

You also need to get plenty of exposure to light. Light is necessary for serotonin production. Get some natural sunlight each day, or consider buying a light box.

Finally, any food that is rich in minerals, especially calcium, magnesium and silicon, induces a calming action on the mind, while a deficiency can lead to sleep problems. Try to include foods rich in these minerals, such as watercress, broccoli, parsley, leeks, spinach, almonds, sesame seeds, sunflower seeds, dried figs, pulses, beans, lentils, brown rice, peaches, bananas, dates, avocados, raisins and sea vegetables.

STEP TWO: GOOD SLEEPING HABITS

- Stick to a regular sleep-wake pattern, even on weekends. Ideally you should aim to be in bed for around 11 p.m., as studies show that people who get to sleep before midnight tend to wake more refreshed than those who go to bed in the small hours.
- Decide how much sleep you need. Eight hours is enough for most people, but you may need more or less to feel alert and refresh. If you want to nap during the day, research shows that 25 minutes is the optimum amount of time for a refreshing nap.
- Make sure your mattress and bed are comfortable. Use your bed only for sleeping and sex, that way you'll associate it with rest and pleasure. Block out noise and light (light impairs the production of melatonin). Sleep in a well-ventilated, cool but not cold room as your body temperature naturally falls during the night.
- Wind down for an hour or so before you go to bed. Activity delays melatonin production. Try taking a nice bath, doing yoga, having a quiet chat, making love, doing relaxation exercises or drinking a cup of chamomile tea. If you can't sleep after lying in bed for more than half an hour, get up and do something monotonous like reading or ironing. Then, when you feel sleepy, go to bed.

- It isn't wise to eat a heavy meal or drink a lot before night time. Stay away from caffeine. Alcohol isn't a good idea either.
- You might want to add aromatherapy oils, such as lavender or bergamot, to your pre-bed bath. Dead Sea Salts, which contain potassium and magnesium, can have a therapeutic effect on body and mind. Or you can sprinkle a few drops of lavender essential oil on your pillow, or have a gentle massage with lavender or bergamot oils. Joanna Levett, an aromatherapist who treats women with PCOS, suggests this bath blend to relieve stress and encourage relaxation:
  - 3 drops mood-soothing Neroli
  - 3 drops sedative Lavender
  - 3 drops calming Basil
- Herbs can also help with sleep problems. Valerian, hops, passionflower, chamomile and skullcap all work as gentle sedative and can improve the quality and duration of sleep. White chestnut Bach Flower Remedy calms the mind and instils an air of tranquillity.
- Many women take magnesium tablets to help them sleep better. Magnesium is often called nature's own tranquillizer.
- Try acupressure. There's an acupressure point on your body called heart 7 whose main action is to calm the mind and alleviate insomnia. Trace your little finger down the inside of your wrist to the crease; this is where heart 7 is located. Gently rub the point using your thumb for around 1 minute. Breathe deeply while you do this and feel peace and tranquillity flowing into your body and mind.
- Practise some relaxation techniques. Try lying on your back in bed, tensing every part of your body in turn and then relaxing. This way you can feel how good it is to relax. You might want to do this to the sound of some relaxing music.

- An hour before you go to bed, write a 'to do' list for the next day, put out the clothes you want to wear. This will stop you from mulling over what you need to do and wear tomorrow.

If none of the above works, try not to get upset. Keep things in perspective. The more you worry about not sleeping, the less likely you are to sleep well. And chances are that if you sleep badly one night you'll sleep like a log the next, especially if you're doing your daily exercise.

COPING WITH THE STRESS OF INFERTILITY

If you're having problems getting pregnant, this can be one of the most difficult and stressful things you'll ever face. It can call into question the most basic expectations you have for yourself, your body and your relationship. Acknowledging this is a key to coping. It's normal to feel a monumental sense of loss, to feel stressed, sad or overwhelmed. Don't give yourself a hard time for feeling these things. Allowing yourself to feel these powerful emotions can help you move past them. Couples who are successful in their careers can have a particularly difficult time dealing with the loss of control that comes with not being able to conceive. If you've planned everything – the job, the house, the holidays – and suddenly aren't able to have a child, it can be very hard.

Although the great majority of women with PCOS can and do get pregnant, what follows is designed to help you cope with the infertility roller-coaster of emotions. It's also important you ask your doctor or fertility specialist for advice about how to cope. They may refer you to a specially trained infertility counsellor.

First of all, don't blame yourself. Faced with infertility it's normal to think things like, 'I shouldn't have waited so long,' 'I'm being punished for having that abortion,' 'I should have lost more weight' or 'I should have taken better care of my health.' Self-doubt is a common, but destructive pattern. Dr Yakov Epstein, author of *Getting Pregnant When You Thought You Couldn't*, says people can get caught in negative patterns of thinking that only make things worse. 'Instead of berating yourself,' he says, 'you need to look forward to how you and your partner are going to manage the situation.' When you start feeling like you 'should have' or 'could have' done things differently, remind yourself that infertility is *not your fault*. Even if you could have made different decisions in the past, they're behind you now. Look forward.

Educate yourself about infertility: Read, read, read and ask questions. This is solid advice when you face any problem, but it's especially important when dealing with infertility or subfertility because the technology is complicated and changes so quickly. 'You've got to understand what's happening medically,' says Dr Epstein, 'or you won't be able to make informed choices.'

Work as a team with your partner. Don't give in to the temptation to blame each other. Instead, help each other. This doesn't mean you need to feel the same thing at the same time, but it does mean paying attention to what your partner is going through. This is crucial. If you're taking care of each other emotionally, you can unite to fight the problem. Practical issues can also help you work with, not against, each other. If you're undergoing treatment, he can take on the household duties. Or if you need hormone injections, he can administer them. Work together to find ways to share the burden, so each of you carries less of it.

- Say 'No' to baby-focused activities. If certain gatherings or celebrations are too painful for you, give yourself permission to avoid them when you're having a particularly tough time. To avoid hurt feelings send a present instead, advises Alice Domar, a psychologist who specializes in helping couples with fertility problems.

- Get support from professionals or other infertile couples. Because society often fails to recognize the grief caused by infertility, those affected tend to hide how they feel, which only leads to feelings of shame and isolation. Finding other people who are going through the same thing, or talking to people who work in the field of infertility, can help you see that you're not alone. One study of women undergoing IVF found that those who openly discuss their emotions have a higher pregnancy rate than who don't. Find a support group through CHILD (the UK's National Infertility Support Network) so you can link up with other couples in your situation.

'I can't tell you what a relief it was to be able to talk to other couples who knew exactly what it was like for us. I'd say it was one of the main things that helped us cope.'
Charlotte, 33

- Take care of yourself by pursuing other interests. While being treated for infertility can feel like a full- or at least part-time job, it's important to keep up with some of the activities or hobbies that bring you pleasure. It won't be easy especially if you're doing something like going in for a blood test every other day, but look for ways to take care of yourself. Get a massage, have a manicure – anything that can give you relief from the focus on fertility.

- Decide how long you're going to carry on trying. You can't go on with treatments for ever – the strain would be too much. There are other options out there you can consider, such as adoption or fostering. Considering these options can give you incredible peace of mind, because in one way or another you can become parents.

- Decide how much you're willing to pay. Infertility treatment can be an expensive business. As from April 2005, couples in which the woman is aged 23 to 39, and who have been trying for a baby for two years, will be offered at least one free cycle of IVF treatment. And while every couple has the right to be assessed for treatment on the NHS, not all couples will be deemed eligible for treatment. You may also find that what is available to you is rationed. If you decide to seek treatment privately – or, as many couples do, use a mix of both NHS and private treatment – always ask in advance what the full cost of each treatment cycle is likely to be. Don't forget the hidden costs, too, of taking time off work and travel expenses – you may need to make many journeys to the clinic.

- Once you know how much your treatment is likely to cost, agree with your partner how much money you're prepared to or can afford to spend in total. If your first round of treatment doesn't work, could you afford another? And possibly another? Having a baby may be a priceless gift, but pushing yourselves into financial ruin will only add to the stresses you already face.

- It may seem hard, but whether you end up with children or not there are opportunities for growth and fulfilment. Having a child is a wonderful and precious experience, but it isn't the only wonderful and precious experience out there.

CHAPTER 16
COPING WITH DEPRESSION AND LOW MOODS

PCOS can be frightening, frustrating and overwhelming. Anxiety about your appearance, grief about loss of control over family planning and anger at years of misdiagnoses are all common. When you add to that fears about the elevated risk of life-threatening medical conditions in the future and the side-effects of medication, it can seem hopeless. Small wonder women can suffer depression as a side-effect of PCOS, or feel depressed because of PCOS-related difficulties.

We don't know yet if depression is a symptom of PCOS or whether the PCOS symptoms such as weight gain and infertility cause depression. But one thing is clear from PCOS research:[1] PCOS can and does have a negative effect on mood, libido, health and well-being. In this chapter we'll be looking at ways you can deal with low moods and depression so you can keep going with your self-help plan.

Depression, stress and anxiety can manifest themselves in physical symptoms such as insomnia, headaches, fatigue, sudden loss or increase of appetite, emotional symptoms such as feelings of sadness, hopelessness, emptiness or guilt as well as behavioural changes like poor concentration, loss of libido, memory loss and withdrawal from social interaction.

Don't forget, though, that there are also other types of depression which may have nothing to do with your PCOS, such as postnatal depression after the birth of a child, reactive depression after the loss of a job or the end of a relationship or a bereavement, seasonal affective disorder, which comes from a lack of natural sunlight, and biochemicial depression as a result of chemical imbalances in the body, sometimes due to a nutritional deficiency or a genetically inherited condition. Some people even experience depression as a result of an allergic reaction or food intolerance, the most common being to wheat and dairy products.

SELF-HELP

Since PCOS often strikes at the heart of our femininity and focuses attention on our appearance, the chances are your self-esteem isn't as solid as it could be. And when self-esteem is poor you're far more likely to experience low moods or depression. There are some great techniques, however, that you can use to counter negative feelings about yourself.

A POSITIVE LITTLE VOICE

If you analyse your thoughts you may be surprised how negative they are. For example, if you drop something you may think, 'Gosh, I'm stupid.' If you bump into someone you may think, 'Why am I so clumsy?' and so on. If you're struggling with your weight you may think, 'I'm fat and ugly.'

Try to catch yourself every time you have a negative thought about yourself or the things you do – and counter that thought with one that is more positive, and yes, more realistic. If you drop something or make a mistake, try: 'OK, I messed up, but what about all the times when I've got things right?' or 'I was looking where I was going, the other person wasn't,' and if you feel very brave go for, 'That wasn't my fault.'

MAKE A LIST

List all the good things in your life. They could be such things as a job you enjoy, a loyal friend, a fascinating hobby, your dog, the trees in your garden and so on. Now make a list of all the good things in yourself. Have a good think now, as there's bound to be a lot more than you realized. You might be a good listener, or a great poet or have a great sense of humour.

ACCEPT WHAT YOU CAN'T CHANGE

Some things in life simply can't be changed. For example, if you're tall or short there's not a lot you can do about it. Neither can you change the fact that you've got PCOS – although as we've seen in this book there are many, many things you can do to improve the situation. Acknowledging what you cannot change is fundamental to happiness, for in accepting things as they are and trying to live with them in the best way you can, you let go of a great deal of frustration.

FIND NEW CHALLENGES

Taking on a new challenge can be incredibly rewarding and can make you feel more positive about yourself. If you've always wanted to learn how to play the piano, book some lessons. Consider taking up painting, singing, jewellery-making, writing – the list is endless. Or perhaps you might like to get some new qualifications or take up a course or even a subject that is helpful with dealing with PCOS such as homoeopathy, reflexology, massage and so on.

GET ACTIVE

Physical activity can contribute to a sense of well-being.[2] In fact, regular exercise is considered by some experts to be one of the most effective treatments for countering depression. Plan to have at least 30 minutes of gentle exercise a day.

EVERYDAY BOOSTERS

Sing along to your favourite music, have a good cry to release excess stress, and have a good laugh. Laughter sends chemicals called endorphins whizzing around your body to make you feel naturally high. So do something to get you chuckling, from watching a funny film to calling an old friend.

FOOD AND YOUR MOOD

Within the brain, chemicals help transmit messages from one nerve cell to another. There are two such substances that seem to affect our moods: serotonin and norepinephrine. The body makes these endorphins from the foods you eat, and therefore you can, to a certain extent, raise the level of these substances in the brain by eating specific foods. According to depression expert Simon N. Young of the Department of Psychiatry at McGill University in Montreal, low serotonin levels often equal psychiatric symptoms. Studies have shown that getting more serotonin into the brain or stimulating serotonin activity can relieve depression.

The main source of endorphins is sugary and carbohydrate-rich food. This is why you may feel happier when you've eaten a bar of chocolate, a cake, biscuit, white bread with jam, or rice pudding. The problem with this is that these foods, as you know, cause a sudden influx of sugar which leads not just to a rush in serotonin but a rush of insulin, too. Insulin breaks down the sugar quickly, leading to a drop in both sugar and endorphin levels. This leaves you feeling even lower than you did before. To avoid blood sugar swings it's best to eat a healthy diet, like the one outlined in Chapter 6.

Serotonin and norepinephrine are not only made from sugary and starchy foods, however; they are also made from tryptophan and L-phenyl alanine, amino acids present in certain protein foods. Some experts suggest that we take supplements of endorphin-producing amino acids, but this can lead to stomach upsets and diarrhoea unless you take a personalized prescription from a nutritional therapist. And don't forget that exercise and sex with a loving partner release endorphins, too!

THE MIND MEAL

The Mind Meal is one practical example of how food can be used to lift mood. It was launched in 2000 and continues to get positive feedback from people who try it.

The Mind Meal consists of the following three courses:

1. Wheat-free pasta with pesto and oil-rich fish
2. Avocado salad and seeds
3. Fruit and oatcakes dessert.

The recipe below serves two hungry or up to four not-so-hungry people. Preparation time shouldn't be more than 30 minutes and all the ingredients are available at your local supermarket or health food store.

WHEAT-FREE PASTA WITH PESTO AND OIL-RICH FISH

250g/9oz packet of wheat-free pasta such as corn and vegetable pasta shells
100g/4oz pesto sauce
170g/6oz tin salmon or other oil-rich fish (mackerel, herring, sardines, pilchards or fresh tuna)

1. Cook the pasta in boiling water per instructions on the packet.
2. When the pasta is ready, drain and transfer to a warmed serving dish. Add approx. 1 tablespoon pesto sauce per person and gently mix with the pasta.
3. Open the tin of fish, drain liquid, remove or crush any large bones and flake with a fork. Add to serving dish and mix gently together.

AVOCADO SALAD AND SEEDS

250g/8oz bag mixed lettuce or 80g/4oz bag watercress
1 avocado
handful (25g/1oz) sunflower seeds
handful pumpkin seeds

1. Place the mixed salad in a serving dish.
2. Remove skin and stone from avocado. Cut avocado into small pieces and add to mixed salad.
3. Sprinkle on the seeds.
4. Serve with olive oil or the salad dressing of your choice.

FRUIT AND OATCAKES DESSERT

2 bananas

2 apples

8 dried apricots

water

8–12 oatcakes

40g/2oz walnuts, chopped

1. Peel the bananas and rinse the apples and dried apricots.
2. Cut the fruit into small pieces, remove the apple core and place together in a small saucepan.
3. Add a minimum of 3 tablespoons of water and simmer gently for 10 minutes or until the fruit is soft, adding more water to prevent the mixture becoming too dry and sticking to the pan.
4. Arrange oatcakes in the bottom of individual bowls (you may have to break them to make them fit).
5. When fruit is soft, pour into individual bowls to cover the oatcakes. If the fruit mixture contains enough liquid the juices will soak into and soften the oatcakes.
6. Serve with a sprinkling of chopped walnuts.

What the Mind Meal doesn't include is just as important as what it does. You won't find artificial additives or added sugars or stimulants. You will also avoid foods like wheat and milk, which can trigger food allergies. What the meal does provide are foods containing valuable vitamins and essential fats, important for emotional and mental health. The oil-rich fish, as well as providing vital Omega 3 essential fatty acids, is also a source of tryptophan. Tryptophan is the essential 'good mood' protein also found in avocado, seeds, dried apricots and walnuts. Absorption of the tryptophan is assisted by the carbohydrates contained in the dessert. The tryptophan is converted into the mood-enhancing brain chemical serotonin, and the banana and avocado also provide some ready-made serotonin. Because the meal has a medium to low GI it will provide a slow release of energy to keep you feeling good for longer.

VITAMIN AND MINERAL DEFICIENCIES

Deficiencies of the B vitamins and vitamin C are most commonly associated with depression. It's a chicken-and-egg situation. Deficiencies can lead to a low mood, but a low mood can also lead to lethargy and lack of interest in preparing good food. Good food sources of vitamin B include milk, yoghurt, cheese, butter, eggs, fish, wholegrain cereals and wheatgerm, dark green vegetables such as broccoli, asparagus and spinach, yeast extract (e.g. Marmite), nuts such as brazil nuts and walnuts, beans, fresh orange juice and bananas. The main sources of vitamin C in our diet come from fresh fruit and vegetables. Fruits high in vitamin C include oranges, strawberries, kiwis, grapefruit, lemons, blackcurrants, rosehips, melon and papaya. Rich vegetable sources of vitamin C include spinach, Brussels sprouts, cabbage, leafy greens, cauliflower, red and green peppers, tomato juice, potatoes, green peas and asparagus.

A zinc deficiency has been noted in some people with depression.[3] This mineral is also essential for healthy reproductive function. Good food sources include shellfish (oysters, mussels, crab and lobster), tinned sardines, turkey, lean red meats such as lamb, hard or crumbly cheese like Cheshire, and wholegrain cereals.

Melvin Konner, MD of Emory University notes that new studies on brain physiology support caffeine's use as a mild anti-depressant. He sees nothing wrong with this if the depression is mild and doesn't need medical attention. We know that with PCOS too much caffeine can wreck your mood, disturb your sleep and rob you of essential nutrients. So if you can't live without it, have no more than one or two cups of tea or coffee a day.

Some studies suggest that chocolate can influence levels of the serotonin, but you're unlikely to eat enough too make much difference, according to Dr Peter Rogers, a psychologist at the University of Bristol. Chocolate probably boosts mood because from an early age we've viewed it as a treat. Again, it's best to eat chocolate only once in a while.

Strange as it seems, many investigators have found that garlic not only has positive effects on blood and cholesterol but that garlic-eaters also experience a decided lift in mood. Hot chilli peppers can produce a similar effect. Might be time to make yourself a curry!

The Mental Health Foundation and food campaign group Sustain claim that changes in eating habits and farming methods over the last 50 years may be responsible for the increase in cases of depression, schizophrenia, attention deficit hyperactivity disorder (ADHD) and Alzheimer's disease. One of the most important findings of the report was a drop in intake by most people of Omega 3 fatty acids.

But the report says that it's not only what we eat, but how it's produced that can also harm our health. Due to changes in the way food is made and manufactured, the amount of essential fats, vitamins and minerals have been reduced and the balance of nutrients has been disturbed.

During the last 50 years the British population has gradually eaten less fresh produce and more saturated fats and sugars, all of which is said to be taking its toll on physical, as well as mental health. Dr Andrew McCulloch, chief executive of the Mental Health Foundation, said that although more research was needed into the effects of food on the brain, the risk of poor health as a result of unhealthy eating habits couldn't be ignored.

Sustain and the Mental Health Foundation have urged people to adopt healthier diets, eat more fresh vegetables, fruit and fish and have also called on the UK Government to increase awareness of the link between poor diet and poor health.

COMFORT EATING

Many of us turn to food for comfort when we feel low or emotional. For some of us, the need to eat sugary foods can be a result of our insulin metabolism being out of synch, in the same way for people with diabetes. (For ways to deal with sugar cravings see page 190.) But sometimes we can turn to unhealthy food as a way of dealing with difficult emotions. If this is you, you need to find ways to stress-proof your diet against comfort eating to help you at those times when you know you're most vulnerable and when you need to adapt your eating to life's routine stressors (work deadlines, rush hour, family dinners, colds, etc.)

PLAN AHEAD

Make out healthy shopping lists, keep healthy snacks on your desk at work and in the cupboard at home, and find out which local restaurants serve healthy foods so you can meet friends there.

Sometimes, however much you plan ahead, things change. You have to be able to adapt your eating routine to our fast-paced society. Keep your cupboards well stocked with emergency healthy foods like soup, beans, tinned veggies and low-fat frozen meals. Fresh fruits and vegetables make great sandwich-fillers and are good to nibble on whenever you feel hungry. If you find your routine totally disrupted, keep as active as you can and help yourself to fruit, yoghurt and made-to-order sandwiches rather than high-fat alternatives.

DON'T SKIP BREAKFAST

This will just make you eat too much later in the day. Plan a mid-morning snack for around 3 hours after breakfast – ideally a protein source like yoghurt and a piece of fruit. Eat your mid-afternoon snack about 3 hours after you eat lunch. This could include protein as well as carbohydrates and be low in fat. Examples include soup with crackers, cottage cheese and fruit, yoghurt and fruit.

EMOTIONAL TRIGGERS

Plan ahead for your emotions. When emotions push you to the fridge, try these quick fixes.

If you're feeling ...	Here's what to do
Happy, excited or proud	Talk about it with someone
	Go do some physical activity with friends
	Go to the gym with a co-worker
	Buy yourself a small gift
Relaxed or content	Take a quiet walk
	Read a favourite book or magazine
	Listen to your favourite music
Sad, discouraged or lonely	Rent a feel-good movie
	Tell a friend or relative that you'd like a hug

If you're feeling ...	Here's what to do
Sad, discouraged or lonely	Call a friend or co-worker to go for a walk with you
	Do something nice for someone else
	Write in your journal
	E-mail a long-lost friend or log on to a PCOS support website
Nervous, worried, stressed or overwhelmed	Take a deep breath, hold it for 10 seconds, and then slowly exhale. Repeat 3 times.
	Talk with a friend
	Do some stretching exercises or take a yoga class
	Write down the situation you're stressed about and make a possible solutions list
Tired	Take a nap
	Do something relaxing
	Do something that you enjoy and doesn't require too much energy
Bored	Take up a new hobby
	Read a magazine
	Go to the gym
	Go for a walk with a friend
	Listen to an interesting radio programme
Angry or frustrated	Blast the stereo and sing or dance like Jennifer Lopez or Bruce Springsteen
	Explain the reasons for your frustration or anger to someone
	Exercise with a friend
	Do some housework

Finally, have a little of what you fancy. An occasional sweet, cake, chocolate or piece of fresh white bread won't hurt. Sometimes these things can cheer you up. A glass or two of wine may be just what you fancy. So go ahead and enjoy it. Remember, everything is good in moderation; just don't get into the habit of turning to alcohol as the only way to relax. The same applies for tea, coffee and chocolate. As long as you're eating the good stuff daily, it really isn't terrible if you eat the not-so-good stuff once in a while. If you're giving in to temptation regularly because you're regularly having crappy days, you need to rethink your life as well as your diet.

Here are some great tips from women we've talked to over the years about stress-proofing your diet against comfort eating:

'Ever since mom gave us a cookie for being good, we've associated food with rewarding ourselves. It's hard to change that mindset, but if you weigh that against a lifetime of being overweight, unhealthy and tired, the decision to change becomes easier. You may want to see a therapist who can help you to learn to nourish your soul rather than fill your stomach.'

'Calling a friend, taking a walk, eating a piece of fruit or something healthy has helped me some days.'

'Try talking back to the little voice and suggest alternatives, such as a hot bubble bath with candlelight, music, and a small glass of wine … reading … shopping (this could be dangerous) or doing something creative.'

'I make myself drink a large glass of water before I eat anything. Many times, after I drink the full glass, I end up not wanting to eat anything because the water has filled my stomach.'

'I would like to suggest exercise – like a kick-boxing class or some type of a high-intensity aerobic class. This kind of class can clear your mind and help you forget about craving something.'

'I tell myself to wait 5 or 10 minutes before I can go get the chocolate bar. By the time I can officially have the candy, I no longer crave it as madly.'

'In your journal, talk with your urge. It will say a host of crazy things. But let it speak. Let it go on and on. Ask it questions. Most of the time it just runs out of steam. But the point is to hear it out. The food shuts it up, but allow your urges to be heard and understood.'

'Just a silly little thing I do, but added to the other suggestions it helps me. I pretend I'm someone I admire – either fictional or real. How would they handle it? Scarlett O'Hara wouldn't let herself pig out on ice cream.'

'No food is illegal … what's wrong is when you eat but your body isn't hungry and calling for food. Remember that grocery stores are open 24 hours a day. Food is all around. There will never be a time when you cannot get to it. So don't feed your soul with things that won't satisfy and leave you hungrier than before.'

'If it's nice weather and still daylight, go to a park and swing on the swings, or just watch the kids doing it. Just go have fun. And just because you had a bad day at work doesn't mean the rest of the day is shot. Tell yourself, "I may have had a bad day up to this point, but I'm not going to let it ruin the rest of my day."'

HELP FROM YOUR DOCTOR

Everybody, whether they have PCOS or not, gets low from time to time, but if you feel that you're not coping and this isn't just a low mood, make sure you seek professional advice from your doctor.

Depression can be treated many ways. Often talk therapy with a professional counsellor can help. Prescription antidepressants are also frequently used to treat depression. Prozac is the most talked about antidepressant but there are many other anti-depressants which your doctor may prescribe you, along with instructions on how much to take and for how long. There are no specific antidepressants used for women with PCOS but it's highly likely that you and your doctor will have to experiment with various medications before you find what works best for you.

NATURAL THERAPIES

ST JOHN'S WORT

There are many brands of St John's Wort on the market which can vary in strength and potency. An overview of 23 clinical trials into St John's Wort and depression was carried out by Klaus Linde and colleagues and published in the *British Medical Journal*, declaring Hypericum extracts to be 'significantly superior' to placebo and indeed, 'similarly effective' to standard antidepressants. Reported side-effects include nausea and extra skin sensitivity, but unlike many antidepressant drugs, St John's Wort hasn't been found to lower sex drive or impair the ability to experience orgasm.

A dose of 900mg of an extract of St John's Wort daily has been shown by studies to be effective in counteracting mild depression. However, the over-the counter preparations are 300mg of extract. Visiting a registered medical herbalist for a tailor-made prescription is another way to make sure you're getting the correct dose. For more information see Chapter 9.

HOMOEOPATHY

Qualified homoeopaths will work out the best treatment for you according to your individual emotional and physical makeup. However, common remedies include Aurum if you feel worthless and self-esteem is low, Ignatia if depression follows deep grief or a failed relationship, and Pulsatilla if you feel emotional and need a lot of reassurance.

Bach Flower Remedies are homoeopathic preparations made from flowers which deal specifically with emotional well-being. Gorse can be used for a sense of hopelessness, Mustard for depression which has no identifiable cause and Honeysuckle for people whose thoughts keep turning to happier times in the past.

AROMATHERAPY

Joanna Levett, an aromatherapist with PCOS who treats women with PCOS, recommends the following bath or massage blend to lift you out of despair.

- 3 drops mood-lifting, feminine Rose
- 3 drops anti-depressant, soothing Camomile
- 2 drops anxiety-relieving Thyme
- Mix with 20 ml carrier oil.

Note:

The above blend isn't suitable if you're pregnant or hoping to be as it can induce periods.

THE POWER OF NOW

Finally, perhaps the best advice we can leave you with is to try to live in the present. All we really have is the now, and cherishing the moment is infinitely better than letting it slip away worrying about the future. How many times have you worried about Christmas and forgot to appreciate the beauty of autumn?

You may well ask: is it possible for someone struggling with irregular periods, facial hair and acne to master the art of living in the now? The thing you need to consider here is what is your alternative? You could sit brooding about how better life would be if you didn't have PCOS and waste precious time with 'if only'. We've all been there but one thing we have learned over the years as we've come to terms with PCOS is that it's far better to take a walk, have a cuddle, write in a diary, surf the internet, read a fabulous book and get on with things we enjoy. It won't always be easy to lift those bleak thoughts, but once you get into the habit of distracting yourself with the business of living life right here, right now, it will become second nature and you'll feel much happier as a result.

CHAPTER 17
MAKING FRIENDS WITH YOUR BODY

Many women struggle with their body image, and PCOS can intensify those feelings. Symptoms like excess hair growth, hair loss, weight problems, acne, absent periods and infertility can all make it hard for you to feel positive, and can even distort your own visual and mental perception of your body.

To be unhappy with the way you look is a heavy burden that lowers self-esteem and negatively affects all areas of your life. Befriending your body, whether it meets your expectations or not, is an important step towards success, and that single embrace will relieve you of an enormous amount of stress, and free up the energy to persevere and succeed with self-help.

You may never fall in love with the image you see in the mirror, but the two of you can at least be friends, if you can change your mind-set.

BECOME A MEDIA CRITIC

First of all, set a healthy objective for how you'd like to look. Society portrays men's and women's figures that are difficult to obtain. Many women strive to reach goals that are either unattainable or unhealthy. Most beauty magazines are filled with pictures of tall, lean women, while the average British woman is 5'4' and 143 lb (10 st 3) and the average American woman is 5'5' and 155 lb (11 st 1).

The media is full of advertisements, actresses, magazines and fashion models who say 'thin is in'. Most of the models you see today weight 23 per cent less than the average woman. Many women who try to achieve this look will become unhealthy due to excessive dieting and exercise. So many of us look at celebrities as role models. But the women who gleam from the pages of the glossies set up unrealistic and hard-to-sustain goals. They're often gifted with unusual bodies, or have made their bodies that way with unhealthy eating habits, and most are seen in photographs that have been retouched to make them look flawless. Stop sticking celeb pics on your fridge as 'motivation', and avoid reading fashion magazines for a while. Instead, focus on your own personal fitness needs: Find a real woman with PCOS you know whose body you admire and ask her for inspiration on staying in shape.

The best solution to the unrealistic and unrepresentative images of the media is to shut them out. Ask yourself how you feel when you read a fashion magazine or watch a TV advertisement? Chance are you'll be hitting the fridge. Now ask yourself, do I really need to read this? Do I really need to support the industry that creates this? Perhaps you could substitute a different kind of magazine, one that features a wide variety of body shapes.

Radiance in the US is an upbeat, optimistic magazine for real-sized women and now has an on-line version (www.radiancemagazine.com).

As for the adverts, turn the TV off, or use the time they're on to do some stretching exercises or to make a cup of herbal tea. If you can't escape the ads, teach yourself to become a media critic and analyse them objectively for the negative messages they convey.

BECOME AN ACTIVIST

You might want to spread your new media awareness and literacy to others. About Face (www.about-face.org) is a fabulous non-profit media organization focused on the unfair and unrealistic presentation of female images in the media. One of the perks of the website are the great stickers, slogans, posters and T-shirts you can purchase. It's hard to feel bad about your thighs when you're wearing a T-shirt that says 'Goddesses have hips.'

If you're involved in a PCOS support group you might want to ask if the group can spend some time discussing media literacy and activism. Beyond PCOS support groups, you might want to consider starting another type of support group in your area; one that promotes an acceptance of all body types. And don't forget to be an activist at home, too. Take a careful look at your own comments. For example, instead of 'You look great, have you lost weight?' say 'How are you today?' Instead of 'I shouldn't be eating this, I feel guilty', say 'Every now and then I enjoy a good dessert.'

TALK BACK

It's hard to tune out the voices that tell you how you should look, from your well-meaning aunt who regularly comments on your weight to a co-worker who chastises you for indulging in the occasional bar of chocolate. The next time someone offers you a nugget of useless and unhelpful wisdom, speak up. Whether it's a gentle 'Thanks, but I would prefer it if we didn't discuss my diet,' or a blunt 'That was rude of you to say,' standing up for yourself can boost your confidence – while sending the message that you want to be accepted as you are.

GET MOVING

Sedentary lifestyles breed self-criticism. As soon as you get active, you'll begin feeling better about yourself, and eventually you will see results. Once you start exercising, you're going to experience physical and mental benefits – no matter what size you are – as exercise raises levels of the feel-good endorphins, your body's natural hormones that give you a lift. Too self-conscious to strut your stuff at the gym? Get started at home and customize your activity to your personality and interests. Dancing, jogging, swimming – whatever you choose, find the activity and environment that's right and fun for you.

Don't fall into the trap of exercising just for weight loss, though – remember, it can also dramatically improve your mood and self-esteem.

CHANGE YOUR PERCEPTION

Body image is based on perception, and perception can be changed because you're the one in charge of your thoughts. In fact, exciting new research is suggesting that our perceptions of our body may be completely controlled by our mind — and our mind can often be wrong.

Once a perception is changed, it becomes reality. For example: a woman with large thighs can think of them as large and unattractive, or she can think of them as thighs that take her where she wants to go and help her get through her day. A mole can be thought of as unattractive or interesting and adding character.

Examine yourself in a mirror and make a list of all your positive attributes. Everyone can find something they like. Consider not just body parts like your eyes, nose or hair, but also body attributes such as stamina, co-ordination and strength. Shift your focus to the positive and remember that the way you feel about your body is potentially more important to the outside world than anything anyone else thinks. When you feel good about yourself you tend to be more confident, and this leads to more acceptance from others. The next time you meet a new group of people, think about your lovely eyes or winning smile rather than the size of your waist or bottom. The boost you get from this positive focus will create a positive impression on others.

'I practised complimenting my hair and my eyes for a couple of weeks before a friend's party — and people kept asking what I'd changed because I looked so good. All I'd changed was my attitude.'
Shona, 26

SURROUND YOURSELF WITH PEOPLE OF ALL SHAPES AND SIZES

Surrounding yourself with people who accept you for who you are, and not what they would like you to be, will help you accept yourself. These people recognize that our differences are to be embraced and make each of us unique. Also assess your prejudices against people of all shapes and sizes. Do you have an aversion to thin, overweight, or fit people? We all come from different backgrounds and environments, and are all genetically different. Until you have walked in someone else's shoes it's not fair to judge them. Educate yourself so you can dispel myths such as 'large people have no willpower' or 'skinny people are fit and healthy'.

SHARE YOUR CONCERNS

Confide in someone close about your concerns about body image. You may find that they also have concerns of their own. Better still, confide in another women who has PCOS. If, however, you're deeply affected by the way you look it may be best to seek the help of a professional. Your doctor should be able to refer you.

'I was so down about the way I looked that I got up the courage to talk to my sister. I was amazed to find she felt that way too.'
Emily, 21

THROW AWAY CLOTHES THAT DON'T FIT

Holding on to clothes that don't fit you can only remind you that you don't look the same as you once did. This causes you stress and can affect your body image negatively. Do yourself a favour and give the clothes that no longer fit you to someone that can use them. If you can afford to, buy yourself new clothes that fit you and you feel comfortable in now!

STOP WEIGHING YOURSELF

Your weight may fluctuate by 5 or more pounds within a single day or from one day to the next. This weight fluctuation can be caused by water retention, different clothing, weighing at different times of the day, etc. It's very difficult to gain or lose even one pound of fat throughout the course of a day. Gaining and losing fat are slow processes that add up over time. Therefore, weighing yourself after a large meal or exercise, with different scales, or more than once a day isn't a good indicator of fat gain or loss.

READ A SELF-HELP BOOK

This chapter is an introduction to the problem of body image. If you're among the many women with PCOS who feel it's a core issue for you, you may want to study the topic in more detail. There are plenty of popular books on the subject. For girls and women we recommend, Kaz Cooke's *Real Gorgeous: The Truth about Body and Beauty*. We also recommend Thomas Cash's, *The Body Image Workbook*; which boils down his cognitive-behavioural therapy approach to body-image dissatisfaction into eight steps. Both of these books are available from amazon.com.

HELP THE NEXT GENERATION

If you can help one young girl to avoid adopting a beauty-obsessed, body-hating attitude you'll be part of the solution, not the problem. Help your daughters or young girls you come into contact with feel comfortable in their own skins:

Be a role model. Wear your own weight and shape with comfort and pride. Work through your own negative attitudes and your kids will benefit, too.

Take the time to help your teen find a style that looks good on her. No one looks good in everything. You may be at your wits' end standing outside the shop changing room, but resist muttering 'If you'd only lose a few pounds, buying clothes wouldn't be such a chore.'

Stop discussing weight and diets – your own or others' – around teenage girls. The comments of adults, especially mothers, can be powerful contributors to weight and body concerns. If you do talk about food, educate your adolescent about the importance of healthy eating.

Avoid fighting over food. Don't limit portions or ban certain types of foods. But do help your teens learn about nutrition so that they know what their bodies need to stay healthy.

Enjoy your food. Make sure your kids know that eating is one of life's great joys, that satisfying hunger is nothing to be ashamed of.

Encourage your teen to feel comfortable with her body. Draw her a warm bath. Hug her often. After she's had a hard day at school, offer to massage her back.

Don't comment on a teen's weight, or let others comment. Instead, comment on her explosive science project or the superb job she did cleaning her room. You can't have both good self-esteem and a poor body image, so help that self-esteem along.

THE PAYOFF

Taking small steps like these can lead to major improvements in your body image, and increased self-acceptance. Keep on trying – it may take weeks or months before you start to feel better, but cultivating a healthier attitude about yourself paves the way for happiness and self-esteem, and your confidence will spill over into your career, your relationships and your determination not to let PCOS rule your life.

CHAPTER 18
GETTING THE EMOTIONAL SUPPORT YOU WANT

The people in your support network need to know how you are and what PCOS is, as well as how you feel about it, so that in times of high emotion when you feel like giving up they can be gently supportive and encouraging and won't say or do things that will make you feel worse because they don't understand.

HELPING FAMILY AND FRIENDS UNDERSTAND THE CHALLENGES YOU FACE

Try to be honest and direct with those you care about. Remember, the more people know about PCOS, the less explaining you'll need to do. And the less explaining other women with PCOS will need to do as well.

It often won't be easy to talk about how PCOS makes you feel, so you do need to have a think first about how you want to express yourself. Before describing how you feel to others, spend some time thinking about how you actually do feel. It may be hard for you to admit to yourself that you feel angry, resentful, frustrated, envious, unattractive and so on, but the only way to deal with 'ugly' feelings is to acknowledge them first. Then you can let them go.

When you start expressing yourself to others, try not to make assumptions about how you think they feel or think about you. For example, telling someone 'I know you find it hard to love me because I'm so hairy, fat and spotty,' or 'You know how hard it is for me to lose weight, so why do you keep buying me cakes and sweets?' Such statements seem like accusations and set up a hostile atmosphere that isn't conducive to creating the understanding and support you need.

There are bound to be times when someone upsets or makes things hard for you by doing or saying things that are hurtful. When this happens, have a good long think before you fly off the handle. Perhaps you have misinterpreted the situation. If your mother brings you a box of chocolates it could simply be because she wants to show how much she loves you, not because she doesn't care about how much you weigh.

If you feel slighted or upset, avoid generalizations and accusations; just say how something or someone has upset you. Help those you care about really start to listen as you explain clearly and honestly and fairly things they might not understand.

For instance, if your friend tells you, 'You've put on masses of weight since we were at school together. You've changed so much. Do you remember when we used to swap clothes at university? Don't think we could do that now, do you?' Instead of getting angry, take a deep breath and answer, 'What you just said really upset me. I have put on weight over the years because weight gain is a symptom of PCOS. I am still the same person, though, and I have feelings.'

If a nosey colleague makes a comment about you not having had children yet, you could answer, 'I would love to have children but it isn't always that easy.' This person might then be sympathetic or probe further with, 'Haven't you got a boy friend yet, then?' It might be tempting to get angry, but that would give the other person the upper hand. Far better simply to say, 'This is something very personal to me and I really don't want to discuss it with people I don't know very well.'

Ideas for boosting your self-esteem (Chapter 16) will help here.

PCOS IS A FAMILY AFFAIR

If you have polycystic ovary syndrome, you already know that you have an increased risk of developing cardiovascular disease, obesity and diabetes. But did you know that if you have PCOS, your immediate family is also at increased risk?

This has been verified by a number of medical studies.[1] Most recently, a study from Kirikkale University in Turkey showed that 40 per cent of mothers and 52 per cent of fathers of women with PCOS had some degree of glucose intolerance. Parents of women with PCOS had higher levels of insulin resistance than parents of women without the syndrome. A previous study showed that parents of women with PCOS had a higher incidence of insulin resistance and diabetes. Another study, from the Brigham and Women's Hospital in Boston, US, evaluated the sisters of women with polycystic ovary syndrome. These sisters were more obese and had more indications of insulin resistance than sisters of women without PCOS.

Try talking to your parents and siblings about reducing not just your but everyone's risk of developing cardiovascular disease and diabetes. The best way for the whole family to reduce their risk is to eat a much healthier diet, exercise more, and reduce chronic stress, according to the guidelines we've given throughout this book. Family members should support each other in their efforts to get healthier and avoid the disability and heartache of chronic disease.

YOUR PARTNER

If you're in a relationship the chances are you'll crave the understanding and support of your partner most of all. Trouble is, the typical problems faced by women with PCOS are likely to have most impact on your relationship with your partner. It's hard to keep secrets when you're in a close relationship, but who wants to tell their partner they have to shave every day otherwise they'd have a beard? Who wants to tell their partner they might have problems getting pregnant or that they need to take acne medication? At first you might try to hide the symptoms from your partner by locking the bathroom door, but relationships that survive have to be based on honesty.

Some women find opening up to their partner an empowering experience, and the love, support and empathy they get back strengthens feelings of togetherness. In fact, it might come as a relief to your partner to know why you were being secretive about all those visits to the bathroom or doctor, or that your mood swings weren't his fault.

If your partner truly loves you they'll be concerned about your health, both now and in the long term. If babies are on the agenda it will help them cope better if they know what you're dealing with. A tiny percentage of partners may find it all too much and prefer to end the relationship, but all we can say is you're better off without them. The type of person who runs away at the first sign of trouble isn't worth a second thought, and if PCOS didn't end the relationship something else would have done. You deserve better.

BRINGING YOUR PARTNER/FAMILY WITH YOU ON YOUR JOURNEY OF CHANGE

Here's some advice from Alex Cross and Rachel Green, counselling psychotherapists who run a psycho-emotional support group for women with PCOS (see Resources chapter) at St Ann's Hospital, London:

'We always invite family members to the group so that they can see for themselves what their partners/family members are going through. This is really step one on the path to families' understanding what changes are occurring and *why*. However, in our experience there will often be what we would term "secondary gains" to family members in keeping women with PCOS from changing. For example, if the woman in question does all the cooking in the house, and her family are used to the less "healthy" options, she may encounter resistance to changes that are perceived as advantageous only to her. Or, on a deeper psychological level, a woman with PCOS may have a partner who would begin to feel very insecure were she to lose weight and start to feel more confident within herself. Often, we don't realize that there are secondary gains to keeping those around us feeling insecure, but relationships often thrive on tricky dynamics involving doubt and insecurity on both sides.

'To help the families of those with PCOS to embrace rather than resist change, we try to foster an atmosphere of open exchange and information-giving. For example, trying to get a partner to see that the changes are designed to facilitate improved *health*, rather than to help the woman with PCOS to become more independent of their relationship. Talking with families about PCOS and its distressing symptoms can really help all concerned to understand the syndrome and keep fear of change at bay.

'Part of this process lies in the woman with PCOS *communicating* her needs to her family and partner. If it's hard for her always to have to prepare her food separately, then she needs to tell her family *why* it would help for them all to begin to eat healthier food together. It can never be presumed that families just *should* know what we are going through. Promoting an atmosphere of open and honest communication whilst undergoing change can protect all involved from unnecessary hurt or confusion.'

It's important when you start out on any journey to make preparations and to plan, and a lifestyle change is no different. It's essential to discuss it with your supporters (family, partner, friends), anyone who may be affected by your change.

If they have reservations about the changes that you're making, for example, if it means more work for them, it's often helpful to discuss the potential benefits for them.

For example, many people find that when they reduce intake of refined carbohydrates, they become more even tempered, headaches reduce and energy is steadier, which could lead to an improvement in quality of family life. There's of course the ultimate goal too, of enjoying a longer and healthier life with them.

It's also helpful to explain to them how important it is to you that they are onboard and supportive of your efforts.

Remind the people close to you how important they are to you and thank them for their support as you go along with your journey. Praise works far better than criticism, and is how you want to encourage yourself along the road too.

WHAT IF THEY DON'T LIKE IT?

It might be difficult to face but some supporters may be interested in keeping you as you are. Indicators of this may be deliberate attempts to sabotage your efforts, such as buying you chocolates for doing so well with your new healthy lifestyle this month. Once may be a mistake, and you could offer suitable alternative rewards for the future such as some make up or bath indulgences, or a magazine. If it happens repeatedly, you might want to discuss with them why this is happening. If your supporters are clear that they don't like the changes you're making, you could ask why they don't want you to feel better in yourself? Reasons can range from dislike of change, which is usually caused by a fear of losing you, to jealousy, which may also have a fear element. If it causes difficulties with your partner, consider professional help from an organization such as Relate which can help you to discuss what you're both feeling and to communicate more clearly in future.

Generally, you may have to educate them that you have a right to change and develop and that this is how it's going to be in future. For children, this can be a useful positive model of how people continue to evolve throughout their whole lives, and that choosing to make a change is very possible. Bear in mind if family members do complain initially that people usually adjust and relationships can actually be stronger for having got through it together.

If one of your supporters gives you an ultimatum about the lifestyle changes you're making, you may need to consider whether you want to continue to have such people around you.

SEX

Whether you're in a relationship with a partner or not, sex matters. If you're single you need to be feeling good about sex, but that isn't always easy if you've got PCOS. When relationships are just beginning it's only natural to try and hide anything that might appear to be less than perfect, especially excess facial hair and acne, and perhaps areas of your body that you feel uncomfortable with. Chances are before every date you spend hours removing any sign of PCOS, carefully applying make up and thinking long and hard about which outfit will flatter you most. Trouble is, it's impossible to keep this up as the weeks turn into months, and if the relationship is serious your partner will start to find out more about you. Once again we think it's really important at this stage in the relationship that you're honest and open about PCOS and the unique problems you face.

⇨ SEX 'KEEPS YOU CALM'

Having sex before speaking in public could be one way of beating stage fright, a report has claimed. During studies to assess the effect of sex on nerves, University of Paisley psychologist Ian Brody found that people who have penetrative sex before appearing in public are less stressed and perform better. And the effect could last for up to a week.

Whether your relationship is in the early stages or you have been together for years, women with PCOS can and do experience loss of libido. It's not usually sex itself they dislike, but their own bodies, and this can lead to inhibitions. We've talked to many women with PCOS who feel so unattractive that they won't allow their partners to see them naked.

The problem with this is if you feel inhibited and recoil from physical intimacy, your partner may start to think you're no longer in love with him or that you don't find him physically attractive. If, however, you have the courage to say you don't want sex because you feel insecure about your appearance, you may find that your partner feels enormous relief that he isn't the cause of the problem. He may even tell you that he still thinks you're attractive. If he does, don't accuse him of saying this just to make you feel better. It's also important for you to reassure him that you still love him.

Open yourself up to the possibility that true love is about far more than physical appearance, even if that is how the two of you were initially attracted to each other. Accept that your partner loves you for who and what you are, not for the circumference of your thighs So many women let poor body image affect their sex lives. The simple fact is that in the throes of passion your partner won't be checking out your cellulite, and neither should you. A confident woman is much more attractive than one who tries to cover herself up. Whenever you find yourself worrying about acne, a roll of fat or any other perceived shortcoming, channel your interest to the erotic sensations going on – the feel of your skin against your partner's, the emotional closeness between the two of you, how the kisses feel. While it may take effort to refocus your attention during lovemaking, you'll find that the more you do it, the easier it will become over time. You'll feel more sensual, which can lead to a happier and healthier love life.

Remember that wonderful scene in *Bridget Jones: Edge of Reason* when Bridget covers herself up with blankets as she heads to the bathroom after a night of passion because she feels embarrassed to show her curvy bits. Darcy reassures her that he loves every bit of her. Men tend to feel differently than women about curves in any case: oftentimes what we see as flab, they see as sensual and exciting.

If you really can't bring yourself to talk through your issues about sex with your partner you may want to seek the advice of a sex therapist or a relationship counsellor. You might find it easier to talk to an outside party about the problems you have with your appearance, and a counsellor would try to give you the strength and encouragement you need to be able to open up to your partner.

NATURAL WAYS TO BOOST YOUR LIBIDO

PCOS can contribute to a loss of libido but it's important to understand that it isn't the only cause of low libido by far. Common contributors include sexual familiarity/boredom, tiredness, stress, many commonly prescribed drugs, the children, illness, too much alcohol, too much food and too many other things that need to be done. Some of these contributory problems have nothing to do with PCOS and can be worked on to great effect, and a determined effort to put your love life back into a more prominent position on your list of priorities can make a big difference. The following tips might help:

- Work on your self-image. It's hard to feel sexy if you haven't taken good care of yourself. Pamper yourself, treat yourself to some inviting perfume, buy some nice underwear, maybe have a facial, or buy some nice body products. If you think you're looking desirable, you're more likely to be confident and receptive. (See our body image-boosting tips in Chapter 17.)

- Watch your alcohol intake. Two units of alcohol appear to have maximum effect. Larger volumes have the opposite effect.

- Try to get enough sleep. Chronic exhaustion and sexy don't mix.

- Regular, moderately energetic exercise for around 30 minutes a day can help to increase sex drive, as can a healthy diet. If you follow our guidelines in Part 2 for healthy diet and exercise, chances are your libido will bounce back.

- Cut down on smoking, or even better, stop altogether. Smoking reduces oestrogen levels in women and has a long-term detrimental effect on sex drive. In men, smoking cigarettes lowers testosterone levels, and one study showed that the association between quality of erection and the number of cigarettes smoked wasn't a favourable one!

- Check with your doctor that you're not taking medications that are known to reduce libido, and, if you are, ask about alternatives. Drugs that can cause problems include certain heart and blood pressure medications, tranquillizers, anti-depressants, steroids, some anti-histamine pills and some cholesterol-lowering drugs. The oral contraceptive has also been linked to a reduction in sex drive.

- Don't forget that perhaps the most potent sex organ is the brain. So think sexy, imagine sexy, and consider reading sexy or romantic books, or watching sexy or romantic films. It can all help to switch the brain from harassed mode to sexy mode, and every little helps.

REACHING OUT TO OTHERS

PCOS can understandably cause you to focus wholly on your symptoms and your body and what you need, but never forget that relationships are about give and take. In return for the support and understanding of those you care about, don't withdraw into your PCOS bubble. Give that support, understanding and love back in return. For example, hugging your partner will make you feel hugged, too. Phoning a friend who needs a listening ear can give both of you a lift. Showing interest in what's happening with your family can make you all feel loved and involved in each other's lives.

It really doesn't take much. You can make someone feel special and loved with a few carefully chosen words or actions, and it's highly likely that when they get the opportunity they will return the favour. We're not saying that you should give to others in order to get back. What we are saying is if you want to receive love, support and understanding you also have to give, listen, support and understand. That's the first and last rule of relationships that survive the test of time, and survive PCOS.

And reaching out to others with PCOS is another great way to build more support into the equation. If you can share your experiences, ideas and thoughts with women and their families who are coping with the condition, then everything you've learned can do someone else good too. Not to mention giving you the feelgood factor.

CHAPTER 19
TACKLING DEEPER ISSUES – RECLAIM YOUR FEMININITY, YOUR PASSION AND YOUR LIFE

Finding out you have PCOS and discovering what risks there are can bring up a lot of deeper emotional issues. The process of having to re-understand yourself in the light of this condition can make you think about everything from your femininity to your self-esteem, your willingness to embrace change, your visions of yourself as a mother, your fears about mortality, your ideas about your relationship and what you want from it, and your fears about taking responsibility for yourself.

This chapter looks at some of these difficult questions that can come up. You'll find coping strategies designed to help you create a brighter future and a more peaceful, joyous outlook for yourself.

Q:'I FEEL LIKE PCOS HAS CHALLENGED – OR EVEN STOLEN – MY FEMININITY'

There's no denying that PCOS symptoms and fertility issues can make you feel less of a woman. Symptoms like facial hair, acne, knowing you have too much testosterone and weight problems can trigger great insecurities about your femininity. If you're feeling hairy, fat and invisible is it possible to reframe all this so you can celebrate yourself as an individual and a woman?

Following the diet and lifestyle guidelines in this book and working on your self-esteem will help keep your symptoms under control and help you feel better about yourself. The latter is important because when most of us say we want to feel more feminine what we are really saying is we want to feel more confident about ourselves. It will, however, take a few months to see an improvement, so to keep your motivation going in the mean time we've put together the following feel-more-feminine quick-fix tips from women with PCOS. We hope they help you feel more confident, beautiful and feminine.

'If I'm feeling really down on myself, a couple of days of eating healthily and exercising harder makes me feel better and more attractive. When I feel good, I instantly take on confidence.'

'I throw away any clothing that makes me feel bad about myself. Maybe the colour's not right or it clings in the wrong places, but if I feel bad in it twice, it goes in the car boot bag.'

'Lipstick! It's cheap, it's easy and you can carry it anywhere. When I don't have time to put on a full face of makeup, I make do with cover-up, mascara and a flattering slick of lippie. When I do have time to go all-out, lipstick is the finishing touch. I keep a basket of lipsticks and in the morning I pull one out at random. It keeps my look fresh and it's fun feeling I look a little different every day.'

'Apart from diamonds, I think a girl's best friend are shoes. So if I need a pick-me-up, I'll slip on a favourite pair of heels that make me walk nice and tall. I feel confident and sexy, and I'm ready to take on the world!'

'It doesn't matter where I'm going or what I'm doing, I always "dress" my hands. That means I always have my nails shaped and varnished. I finish them off with a touch of oil to keep them healthy and strong. Nice hands are a statement of how I look after myself and — no matter what else I'm wearing — that I am a true girl at heart.'

'I love to take a bath and pour in lovely-smelling bubble bath and oils. I then light a few candles and add a bit of background music and soak until I feel whole again.'

'When I start to get a little down in the dumps and my appearance starts to follow, I get a haircut. It doesn't matter if it's just a trim or a brand new style: it makes me feel like a new woman.'

'I'm a fan of getting a pedicure when I start to feel a bit dowdy. It makes me feel pretty inside and out, and I look better in sandals, too.'

Think back to the last time you felt really feminine. Chances are you were dressed to the nines for a special event. Hair, nails and high heels all perfectly in place. So take simple steps to feel more polished. Unleash that hair from its bobble, paint your nails and, if you're always in flats, make the effort to wear heels at least one day a week. (If you work, take them with you in a bag or leave a pair stashed under your desk.) And what is the point of having beautiful jewellery if you only wear it on your birthday and at Christmas? Get your money's worth and show it off – it will glam up everyday outfits. And try some of these:

- Sign up for some belly dancing classes. The belly dance isn't just a workout or a dance. It's a spiritual experience which will literally transform your personality and make you feel more sensual and feminine.
- If you'd like to reintroduce a sense of femininity to your image, think about what you can wear beneath your clothes to help you feel this way. Pretty underwear adds a sense of femininity. Or try a lacy vest beneath a V-neck jumper to soften its strong lines.
- Keep a note of all the compliments you receive in a month. Jot down everything from the 'Oooh I like your hair style,' to 'Thanks, for doing that, you're really kind.' Then, instead of dismissing them with a 'Yeah, right', take a deep breath and accept them with a confident 'Thank you' and a smile. When you review your list at the end of the month you may be surprised at how often others pay you compliments – on everything from your sense of style to your thoughtfulness and the great way you look in a flattering top or skirt. Seeing them written down all together, you'll start to believe them too.

Here are some practical tips for keeping in touch with your femininity from Alex Cross and Rachel Green, counselling psychotherapists at St Ann's Hospital, London:

'If you can understand symptoms such as hirsutism and acne aren't personal idiosyncrasies, but part of your wider PCOS picture, it can keep you from condemning your physical appearance. Many of our PCOS group attendees have found acknowledging their symptoms publicly in a support group like this really helped them to live with them. I will always remember introducing a group exercise on "hairiness" in the first group and observing a highly charged, animated dialogue occurring between the women, many of whom acknowledged that this was their first ever experience of discussing such a difficult and embarrassing symptom. It's also worth talking to other women generally about body image – all women are subjected to cultural stereotypes of beauty (every woman will have parts of herself that she hates). Another thing that can help you cope with a sense of loss of femininity is to explore your version of what your perfect self might look like. How realistic are you being? Many times we have heard women say "If I could just get back to the size 10 I achieved for six weeks in 1982, I would feel so differently about myself." It's time to promote a more realistic version of how you might feel good about your physicality, to help you reconcile yourself to what *is*, rather than what *might be*, possible.

'Finally, there's more to femininity than external appearance. We looked at what constitutes a "feminine" woman and cited examples of women from the media that the group agreed promoted a feminine type, but without being thin or 'perfect'. So Dawn French and Fern Britton were mentioned a lot, as was Jennifer Lopez's derriere, as examples of women who still appear voluptuous, sexy and feminine. These "alternative" images of femininity seemed to help a lot.'

SEE YOURSELF AS A WHOLE PERSON, NOT A WOMAN WITH PCOS

Try this exercise to help you to view yourself as a whole person, and to encourage you to think of yourself as a whole being, personality and other characteristics in addition to being a woman who has PCOS.

- What words best describe your personality?
- What would your closest family and friends say about you?
- What would your children say about you?
- What would your employer/colleagues say about you?
- What did you do well at school?
- What do you think that you do well? (work, personal, skills, hobbies, talents, etc.)

We are aiming to develop a list of words which describe you, maybe not words you'd use yourself, but those that the people who know you well in different roles (e.g. as a daughter, as a wife, as a mother, as an employee, as a friend) might use to describe you. It's important in this exercise to think only about those who love you and have positive comments for you, as negative comments can sometimes arise where a person has their own problems or issues.

Ask yourself how you'd feel about a friend who had these characteristics.

Now, draw a person (you), and write in these words. Pin this somewhere you will see it to remind yourself of you as a whole person and not just a bag of PCOS symptoms.

IF YOU FEEL YOUR FEMININITY HAS BEEN STOLEN

PCOS is a difficult condition and has been called 'the thief of womanhood' (Kitzinger & Willmott, 2002). But treatments are improving, and in the last 10 years great progress has been made in helping women with PCOS to lose weight, which seems to be the mediating factor for many of the other distressing symptoms. So, it's starting to become clear that appropriate treatment can turn the condition around, and it's no longer an irreversible condition. This is a most important thought to hold onto, because it suggests that you can recover the stolen goods.

If you're experiencing high levels of distress about your PCOS symptoms, here is some advice from Dr Clair Clifford to help you cope:

FOCUS ON THE POSITIVES

Get someone close to you (e.g. a good friend, your mother, your partner) to help you analyse what your best points are (physically). Pick someone who can be fairly honest but not someone who enjoys making you feel bad!

- Think about your face
- Think about your individual features, and body parts
- Think about your body shape
- Think about the way that you dress/your style

As you think about these parts of yourself, identify your best features: you may have beautiful eyes, even white teeth; you may have nice nails or even have a lovely cleavage! Play up the features which work well for you – focus on caring for and enhancing these features, which will make you feel better about yourself.

If you feel very confused about what you should wear to make the best of your particular body shape and features, consider having a style/makeover session with someone such as a personal shopper or one of the many businesses developing to help people with their 'lifestyle'. If you can't afford it, could you ask for this as a gift for birthday or Christmas?

If feeling unfeminine is related to your weight, follow the advice in the next section to give yourself the best chance of success with your attempts to improve your health and improve your body image. If you can nurture yourself, you will do far better at looking after your health than if you try to bully yourself into looking after your health.

If feeling unfeminine is related to fertility problems, please make sure that you follow the advice about giving yourself an optimum chance of having a child in other books such as 'PCOS and your Fertility'. Many women who are having problems conceiving can feel angry towards their bodies, which they see as letting them down. It's important not to let this anger sabotage your attempts to improve your health – it could, for example, make you feel hopeless so that you give up on making healthier food choices.

There are different ways to manage these feelings:

- Keep a diary or journal, where you can record these feelings. The great benefit of a diary is that once written down, it's often easier to let go of these feelings and thoughts. You can use this as much or as little as you like – the book won't mind whether you write daily or monthly or just when steam is coming out of your ears!
- Channel the feelings into some exercise, with obvious associated benefits!
- Talk to someone close, who will understand and let you talk it out. It may not always be your partner, if they feel responsible for the difficulties, or don't want you to upset yourself.

- Challenge any negative automatic thoughts which you might have – these often sneak in and we fail to notice let alone challenge them. They often take the form of thinking in black and white terms, making predictions (guessing) what others think about us and jumping to conclusions, without evidence. A psychologist or CBT therapist can help with this.

GET HELP WITH THE NEGATIVES

If the hair growth is distressing you, research the treatment options and decide which suits your circumstances and your preferences the best. You may be able to receive laser hair removal on the NHS. Similarly, with spots you may need to try several treatments before you find one which is effective and acceptable to you.

If weight or fertility problems are your major concern, look at the different weight-loss methods documented for women with PCOS and work out which *you* could most comfortably fit into your lifestyle. Some dieticians now have a special interest in PCOS, and it may be possible to be referred to someone with such experience for advice.

Plan how you're going to make the changes in your lifestyle, identify when you will find it difficult to stick to the plan and work out solutions for these scenarios. When you have completed this stage thoroughly, you can prepare to start the process. The majority of 'diets' fail because they fall at the first hurdle (e.g. first meal out, first bout of PMS cravings, first time getting late from work starving). So by thinking through when you will find it difficult to stick with it, and planning for those times, you will have a better chance of making permanent changes to your lifestyle and achieving better health. Combine this with an insulin sensitizing drug, which many doctors will now agree to prescribe, and you are giving yourself the best chance of success.

If you find that your concerns about your appearance are affecting your ability to carry out the activities of daily life, or you're having very distressing thoughts about an aspect of your appearance, it may be worth discussing with your GP. There's a condition called Body Dysmorphic Disorder where people become excessively concerned about an 'imagined or slight defect in appearance' which can be helped by psychological therapy.

Q:'WHY ME? WHY HAVE I BEEN LANDED WITH A CONDITION THAT MAKES ME FAT, SPOTTY, HAIRY AND LIKELY TO GET DIABETES? WHAT HAVE I DONE TO DESERVE THIS?'

This is the classic question for anyone dealing with a new diagnosis of PCOS. Your world has suddenly been turned upside down.

The first thing you need to realize is that *PCOS isn't your fault*. As we saw in Part 1 there's a genetic component to the condition, and your genes aren't swappable. Having said this, there's no reason to feel helpless. If you've gained anything from this book we hope it is that there's a lot you can do to manage your symptoms, reduce your long-term health risks and get your life back on track.

Taking an active part in your treatment programme will give you back a feeling of control over your health and your life. A feeling of powerlessness can be overwhelming if you're dealing with a life-long health condition like PCOS which requires visits to the doctor and dealing daily with symptoms, but making positive diet and lifestyle changes can transform those feelings of powerlessness into a more positive outlook.

TURNING 'WHY ME?' INTO 'I AM IN CONTROL'

Alex Cross and Rachel Green have this to say on turning your 'life is so unfair' thinking around:

'The way you think about your PCOS will dictate how able you feel to self-manage the condition. Fact. So if you feel angry and fed up about having PCOS, you're unlikely to facilitate change – and change is a necessary part of effective self-management.

'So how can women with PCOS get over feeling angry that they have the condition? How can they turn their resentment and sense of victimization into a more purposeful energy?

'The route lies in the relationship between self-acceptance and what we call "self-efficacy". If you understand that you have a certain degree of control over symptoms, then you're likely to become more accepting of the condition and more predisposed towards creating helpful changes.

'Take Marie (name changed for confidentiality) as an example. Marie, aged 24, had experienced fluctuating weight for a number of years, coupled with embarrassing hair growth and acne. Having been diagnosed with PCOS as a teenager (but given little information about the condition), she had battled to cope with her distressing symptoms during a critical phase of her development as a woman. She felt really angry that she had PCOS, and internalized a very negative view of herself as a result. She dressed in tracksuits and trainers in order to try and disguise her appearance, and gave out the impression that she "didn't need anyone". This led to her behaving very defensively around other people, who described her as "aggressive" and "unpredictable".

'Marie attended one of our PCOS groups, bringing her mum and boyfriend to the family session. She was able to express her anger in front of her family and they, in turn, were able to understand her struggles more clearly and offer her the support she needed. Marie, through learning about PCOS and her own ability to manage symptoms, underwent quite a visible change throughout the course. She started going to the gym, thinking about what foods she might want to eat, and her appearance began to change. She told us that she felt less "cursed" by PCOS – that she was beginning to accept that she had a health condition and that, by accepting it, she was able to think about the best way(s) of moving herself forward. Her defensive "mask" had noticeably dropped and her mum and boyfriend described her as "calmer", "more chilled out" and "more affectionate"!

'What this case study demonstrates is that empowerment can often fuel greater acceptance. Marie, through gaining information and the support of other women with PCOS, was able to accept her condition. Not only could she accept it (at last) but she could also feel a degree of mastery over her symptoms. In other words, rather than feeling as though PCOS had "descended" upon her as a cruel blow, she was able to view her condition as part of her ongoing identity.

'In our experience, we have been able to change negative thinking around PCOS via a combination of group support (i.e. minimizing isolation) and information to help self-management.

'Finally, in our determinedly optimistic fashion we always try and locate the positives in having a diagnosis of PCOS. What are they? Well, accepting the condition and feeling able to manage symptoms fosters greater self-confidence and sense of personal efficacy. This can enable women with PCOS to lead more purposeful lives within which they feel more in control of their own destiny. Managing symptoms well and living a healthier life helps to protect women with PCOS from all the major health threats such as heart disease and cancer. Not only can you look and feel better, but you can also applaud yourself for becoming an agent in your own health destiny – very empowering and full of feel-good factor!'

CHALLENGING 'WHY ME?' THINKING

'Why me' is one of the most difficult questions which comes up for people experiencing serious health conditions. 'I usually say: "Well, why not you?", and "Why not me, then why not anyone else?"', says Dr Clair Clifford, a psychologist working with women with breast cancer who has PCOS herself. Sometimes we grow up believing that the world is a fair place and that if we do the right thing, nothing bad will happen to us, but unfortunately, real life isn't like this.

Questions like: 'why me?', 'why have I got to cope with this?', 'life isn't fair' often come to mind when someone is frightened and worried that they won't cope. It's all right to have these feelings: after receiving a diagnosis of a serious health condition, such as PCOS, it's common to experience a range of emotions, such as depression, anger, denial and all of these are normal. The difficulty is when these emotions don't pass over and the person is stuck in a position which stops them following treatment advice, or making the lifestyle changes which will alleviate their condition.

We need to identify alternative ways of thinking which will help us to cope. If we feel punished for having PCOS, we will find it harder to make lifestyle changes and to stick to them. If we feel angry about having PCOS, we will find it harder to make lifestyle changes and to stick to them.

If you have a religious faith, sometimes this can help you to cope with these worries. Some people take a more general spiritual approach, and believe that such illnesses may be sent to make us stronger people. Finding a way of thinking which helps you to cope is an individual process, and can vary over time. In the next section I will consider some of the thinking patterns women with PCOS might experience, and how to manage these thoughts:

'I can't cope with this illness.'

'I'm afraid that I'll fail.'

These kinds of thoughts might arise if you don't usually fail at things which you try – you may be very successful at work or in any sphere of your life. But with PCOS, you may feel that the stakes are high in terms of your health or fertility, and the battle is very personal. If these thoughts are troubling you, useful challenges might be to think of your condition as something which you're learning about – On this journey, what is the worst that could happen? Then you will struggle on occasion, but at least you'll know you try, and each 'failure' is an opportunity to learn and to do better the next time.

'What have I done to deserve this?'

PCOS can be a difficult condition to live with because of its links with excess weight, says Dr Clair Clifford. Indeed, the medical advice used to be that symptoms would abate if patients could lose some weight. But that was before it was identified that PCOS women find it harder to lose weight because of the insulin connection. Now there's an acknowledgement that

PCOS women do find it more difficult to lose weight on conventional low-calorie diets. Instead, we are advised to eat in a way which maintains a stable blood sugar level and prevents low blood sugar which triggers excessive insulin release which turns more of the food we consume into fat. The key to this eating is complex carbohydrates and lean protein – essentially low-fat and controlled carbohydrate diets for women who have PCOS.

There's a medical reason why we gain more weight from eating the same food as other people, and this is founded on the insulin connection. There's no need to feel that your eating habits have brought this condition upon yourself – indeed, the last 30 years the medical establishment have focussed on telling us to eat low-fat and low-calorie. We were in effect being told to eat the very foods which turn to sugar in our bodies and mess up our insulin levels.

I think it's safe to say that PCOS is no longer seen as self-induced by over-eating or getting fat, it's actually caused by wrong eating, but exactly what we have been medically advised to do since the 1970s.

Moving on from self-blame, it's also significant that there are now solutions – that there are ways which women with PCOS can successfully lose weight and keep it off, without too much difficulty.

'Change is too hard.'

'I can't change.'

Change can be quite frightening, we are comfortable with things that are familiar and they give us a sense of security. However, once we change our lifestyle, our new behaviours can become as comfortable as our old behaviours were. The key elements to effective change are in the planning, and contingency planning in the preparation process before we put change into place. Just think of the pride you will feel, when you have made the changes and realized your goals.

Today there's a huge amount of support available – via Verity self-help for women with PCOS. But also via web communities which have enabled women with specific concerns (e.g. sticking to a low carbohydrate diet, trying to conceive, etc.) to meet together, support and share.

Q: 'I FEEL SO FULL OF ANGER AND BITTERNESS'

If you've been struggling for years with the medical community or been treated badly/unsuccessfully and feel you have had part of your life stolen from you by PCOS and the lack of a diagnosis/effective treatment, it can be hard not to feel full of rage. How do you combat that?

On a personal level you can get a sense of control back by following the guidelines in this book. You can also channel your rage as a positive energy for change, so that other women don't have to go through what you have. You can become an active part of a support group and dedicate yourself to increasing awareness of the condition. You can work with your GP or local hospital to give talks on PCOS so other women don't have to suffer as you did.

It's understandable to feel angry, but remember that anger can backfire on you, increase your stress levels and trigger symptoms of PCOS. If you can't let go of the anger, channel it into helping yourself and others.

COMBATING SHAME OR DISGUST

Feel the pain and acknowledge the shame that comes with the feelings about your symptoms: PCOS is not pleasant and part of the process is acknowledging the feelings which it produces about ourselves. Write a letter to your critical self telling yourself the damage and pain that your over-criticalness causes. Tell your critical self that you're doing your best and that she should back off! The idea is to vent the frustration and sadness at the illness, and then say how it's going to be from now on. The best position to be in is one where you can nurture your efforts to care for your health, and forgive the mistakes and slip-ups which will inevitably occur.

USE A CUE-CARD

In summarizing some of this work on challenging your negative self-image, it's helpful to develop a cue-card, says Dr Clair Clifford. On this, you can list the situations which trigger negative thoughts about yourself:

Example

Trying on clothes in a high street store -> can't find something you like which fits well -> become demoralized about weight/loss (Thought: I'll never fit into anything fashionable) – feel worthless and weak -> go for a coffee and cake to help me feel better.

The point at which to intervene is when the thought about not fitting into fashionable clothes arises. A cue-card for such situation might read:

'OK, so I can't find anything I like which fits well today, but I am trying my best to follow a healthier lifestyle, and weight loss is known to be difficult for women with PCOS. I will make a choice now to stop looking for today, and maybe I will ask the next larger woman I see whose style I like where she shops, and try to find a more suitable place to go shopping. In the meantime, I want to acknowledge the effort I am putting in, so I will treat myself with a magazine/accessory/makeup which will also make me feel that the shopping trip was worthwhile.'

You can prepare such 'pep-talks' for yourself in advance, as surprisingly many of the situations which weaken our resolve or commitment to our lifestyle plan, arise repeatedly. Here are just a few common ones — you need to work out which are your triggers:

- Being presented with a buffet of lovely looking food at a drinks event or party.
- Feeling very slightly under the weather and considering not going to the gym as you had planned.
- Giving in to just one 'treat' and then giving up on your healthy eating altogether.

The key is to replace your negative automatic thoughts with more balanced, honest and positive statements. Negative thoughts which are triggered by a situation and shaped by our core beliefs about ourselves are dangerous because they lead to depressed and hopeless affect (mood) which decreases your resolve, or makes you give up.

Try to become aware of your negative automatic thoughts and think as if a friend were saying these comments, then talk to yourself as a friend, to find a more balanced view.

Q: 'HOW WILL I EVER FEEL HAPPINESS AGAIN AFTER TWO MISCARRIAGES?'

How can you come to terms with loss and grief and move on without feeling you're forgetting your children, and that living your life isn't an insult to them?

Miscarriage is far more common than you may realize, regardless of whether you have PCOS or not. An estimated one in four women experiences miscarriage, and one in 300 has had three or more.

When you experience a miscarriage you may be surprised by the enormity of your grief. Your loss may feel so painful because there's an immediate psychological and hormonal bonding between a mother and her unborn child.

In an attempt to avoid the pain, many women struggle not to grieve over a miscarriage, but it's vital, for your emotional recovery and growth, to mourn fully such a profound loss. Only when we allow ourselves to feel painful feelings and share our grief with the people we trust are we able to begin the healing process.

Miscarriage is a traumatic experience and you need to treat it with the respect you and your unborn baby deserve. It's crucial that you're kind and nurturing towards yourself at this time, and avoid any situations, such as baby showers, that are going to cause pain. Give yourself the time and space to grieve and to accept and experience all your feelings.

Grief isn't something you can run away from. Symptoms of grief have been observed in women 20 years after a miscarriage. Don't be surprised if you feel a huge sense of guilt and self-blame. It can't be stressed enough that miscarriage isn't your fault, but when you're in pain and desperate to find answers you may well blame yourself or even your doctor or fertility clinic.

Freeing yourself from such negative feelings can add to your sense of closure and may well also contribute to your future happiness and the success of future pregnancies or future fertility treatment, if you decide that is what you want to do. What's more, if you have unresolved grief this may stop you fully experiencing the joy of any future pregnancy. 'If you feel that you have not fully grieved over a miscarriage,' says Niravi Payne, founder of the Whole Person Fertility Program in New York, 'I recommend that you express what you're feeling – verbally or non-verbally – by engaging in some form of grief ceremony.' This can be a funeral or you may also want to write a letter to your unborn child, or say a prayer or record your experiences in a diary. The important thing is to acknowledge your grief. Only then can you move forward.

Q: 'I'M SO SCARED OF DIABETES AND HEART DISEASE – PCOS HAS MADE ME FACE MY OWN MORTALITY AND IT'S FRIGHTENING'

Coming to terms with the dangers of PCOS means you're better equipped to face them – and facing mortality is a difficult thing we all have to do. We hope the following will help you separate PCOS and mortality in your mind and find peace.

It's a sobering thought that PCOS brings with it an increased risk of heart disease, obesity, diabetes and cancer. And yet, although there are without doubt links, heart disease, obesity, and diabetes aren't inevitable results of PCOS. Just as a tall person is more likely to bump their head on a door frame than a small one, not every tall person hits their head on a door, and not everyone with the risk factors gets heart disease or obesity.

Knowing this means you can take action now to protect yourself. Research clearly shows that preventative measures are really effective in cutting your risks. You can stop smoking, you can reduce cholesterol with good eating, you can avoid a couch-potato lifestyle, you can combat hypertension by eating less salt, and you can tackle obesity.

Better still, research also shows that by directly treating PCOS with diet and lifestyle changes, and medication if needed, you can bring your hormone levels into a normal range – not only minimizing or eliminating the symptoms and effects of PCOS, but also cutting the heart disease and cancer risk factors of obesity, high cholesterol and insulin levels. Put simply; altering your diet and lifestyle can help you beat symptoms of PCOS and cut your risk of long-term life-threatening diseases at the same time.

Q:'WE KNOW PCOS MIGHT STOP US HAVING KIDS OF OUR OWN – HOW WOULD I REALLY FEEL ABOUT ADOPTING?'

A big question for couples, and for you – if it does look like getting pregnant naturally isn't likely, how might you approach the adoption option and the emotional adjustments that needs?

The first question you need to ask is do you both feel the same about welcoming a child into your hearts if that child isn't biologically yours? Will you be able to find room in your lives and your hearts for a child, whatever its age or temperament? If you've set your heart on a baby, remember that babies soon grow up and you need to be there as they do, loving and supporting them every step of the way.

The experience of adoption alters your life for ever and can involve feelings of loss, rejection, guilt, shame and grief. Many couples say giving up the hope of a natural birth alters the way they feel about themselves completely. Identifying and acknowledging how you feel can help alleviate some of the feelings of pain, guilt and isolation.

If you both think you'd like to adopt a child, the first thing to do is to contact your nearest adoption agency. You've got the best chance if you're in a relationship and aged between 21 and 35 (40 for the man), but because of the surplus of children with special needs, these rules are becoming far more flexible and there are opportunities even for single women and older couples to put their case forward.

There are no guarantees that you will be matched with a child, and even when everything does fall into place it's still hard work. Adoption isn't for everyone. It has its challenges as well as its joys, and not every couple will feel emotionally equipped to deal with them, but if you do decide to adopt or foster it could turn out to be one of the best and most life-enhancing decisions you ever make.

Q: 'I'VE BEEN IN A PCOS BUBBLE FOR SO LONG – I'M NERVOUS ABOUT JOINING THE REAL WORLD AGAIN'

When you're dealing with an illness it can take up so much of your focus that your horizons shrink down to your daily routine, taking care of yourself and your family, and you don't have time or energy for anything else. Then, finally, as you start to emerge into vitality when your new habits and health become apparent, it can feel odd having the time and desire to go out and do more stuff.

We've both been down the dark PCOS tunnel and we know how hard it can be to face the light again. But we also know that it's possible to connect with fun again, step out of hibernation and into a new life.

Here are some tips from some of your 'soul-cysters':

'Don't wait until you're better at things until you do them. My advice is to just have a go. Half the fun is learning from your mistakes.'

'Be a good role model for your loved ones. Do you want your kids or family or friends to learn confidence or insecurity from you? Let them see you moving forward with optimism, not hanging on to the past.'

'Go through your closet and throw out your old clothes. Are you hanging on to them because of past memories? If so you may find it hard to look ahead because a part of you is stuck in the past.'

'It really is OK to accept all your feelings and not to hide from them. It's OK to feel angry, sad, jealous and all the other emotions you may think of as bad. You can't look to the future unless you acknowledge your feelings and let them go.'

'Don't take yourself too seriously. Get in touch with your childish playfulness and sense of wonder and optimism. Try out new things, shout, laugh and bring everything back into perspective.'

'The recipe for happiness:

Take a couple of good deeds,
a measure of thoughtfulness,
a heaping tablespoon of consideration,
a sizeable portion of forgiveness and mix
thoroughly with tears of joy and seeds of faith.
Blend daily into your life, baked with the warmth of love,
served with a blessing and a smile to make a life full of peace and happiness.
from *A Victorian Grimoire* by Patricia Selsco

Last but by no means least, take time to nourish your soul.

NOURISHING YOUR SPIRIT

Most of us make a list every week of what we need to fill our food cupboards. How about making a weekly 'grocery list' for your spirit as well? Whatever the deeper issues and emotional challenges you are coping with, one of the best ways to increase your resilience is to nurture your soul as well as your body.

Grab a pen and paper and make a list of the things you love, the things your heart and spirit need. A morning set aside to do some gardening or read a book? An hour alone? A long, hot bath? A half-hour to read poetry? A massage? Fresh flowers in your bedroom? A visit to your spiritual home, be it a church, synagogue or a spot in nature that inspires awe in you? A simple meal and heart-to-heart with a close friend? A trip to a museum or art gallery?

On page 345 you'll find some fun tips and exercises for soul-sustenance from other women with PCOS. Make a commitment to your inner self to take time every week for at least one of these things. For true health you need to feed your spirit no less than your mind and body: help yours feel satisfied.

NATURAL THERAPIES THAT LIFT YOUR SPIRITS

Holistic health emphasizes the importance of the whole being rather than the dissection and analysis of individual parts. What comprises the whole being? The body, the mind and the spirit are the basic ingredients to each and every one of us, and for true health all of these need to be nourished and in balance with one another.

There are plenty of natural holistic therapies that can soothe your body, mind and spirit; we've mentioned most of them in this book already. From

Ayurveda to Shiatsu massage, aromatherapy to reflexology, why not ask your friends if they have tried and benefited from any of these, and go for a trial treatment? Or try these life affirming, soul nourishing ideas from other women with PCOS:

'You feel a bit of an idiot the first couple of times, but I recommend belting out your favourite song in the shower!!'
Karen, 26

'Counting the three good things that have happened every day just before going to bed is something I do with my husband each night. It's uplifting to stop and realize that every day has its blessings.'
Carol, 41

'Looking at photo albums always makes me feel good. So many memories to cherish, and so many more to make.'
Laurie-Ann, 28

'Looking in my mobile contacts list and seeing all the people in there who care about me is a real buzz.'
Keisha, 19

'Singing a song with my kids on the walk home from school is great fun and puts all my cares into perspective.'
Anita, 38

'Cooking a Sunday meal and eating it with my family around me is so restorative – especially when they do the washing-up!'

Kate, 38

- Meditation, yoga, and tai chi classes all stress the importance of finding balance and inner peace.
- Massage uses the power of touch to detoxify your body, soothe your mind and uplift your spirit.
- Aromatherapy oils can be very uplifting. Our personal favourites for calm and inner peace are essential oils of lavender, clary sage and sweet orange.
- Plan to escape to the countryside if only for a few hours a week.
- If this isn't possible, take a walk in a park.
- Take time to appreciate the wonders of nature, the colour of the sky, the green of the grass, the birdsong.
- Slow down for a while and enjoy the peace and quiet.

It's surprising how quickly you can restore yourself in these ways. Feeling stressed and below-par is often the result of trying too hard to keep up with the pressures of modern life and neglecting our spiritual side. Take a nature break, enjoy the simple pleasures and restore your self-esteem.

To lead a balanced, healthy, fulfilling life with inner strength we need to be able to stop doing and sometimes just *be*. Just being releases tensions and increases our self-awareness. Spend a few minutes each day in total silence. Turn off the TV or radio. Don't read a book or do anything. This will be difficult at first, but as you get used to it you will be able to do it for longer and be able to balance your being with your doing.

When you spend this kind of time alone, you may feel gratitude for all that you have in life. You may also develop a sense of being at one with the rest of the world and its people, and through this feeling of oneness you may begin to assume more responsibility not just for your health and well-being but for the health and well-being of others and the world you live in.

To feel truly healthy and complete, every woman with PCOS needs to nourish her mind, body and spirit. So whether or not you consider yourself a spiritual person, every time you take time out to dream, to imagine or simply to be, you're taking care of your spirit. This is the real you, and serving it brings you inner peace.

CHAPTER 20
BE INSPIRED BY SUCCESS

Although medications play an important role in controlling your symptoms, there's no doubt that PCOS responds better when you take your health into your own hands. As we've seen throughout this book, there's a lot you can do to minimize the problems associated with PCOS. It may take time and you will need to be dedicated to a healthier way of living, but as the success stories below illustrate, there's absolutely no reason why women with PCOS can't lead healthy, fulfilling and happy lives.

▷ SALLY'S STORY

'After having my period like clockwork until age 20, it stopped altogether for two years. My GP and my gynaecologist told me to simply go on the Pill and it would correct itself. I decided to go off the Pill after about six months and started to see a nutritional therapist. She recommended that I have an ultrasound done of my ovaries after hearing about my other symptoms (irregular periods, inability to lose weight, acne, low body temperature, mild hirsutism, infertility, etc.). Sure enough, in January 2004 I was diagnosed with PCOS. Since then I have been eating a proper diet, exercising and taking supplements such as Vitex, ground flaxseed and homoeopathic remedies.

'Since following this routine I have had the following successes:

- 'Lost 15 pounds (and counting)
- 'Have had a regular period for a year now
- 'Have begun to ovulate
- 'No more digestion difficulties
- 'My skin has cleared up a great deal
- 'My libido has returned (yay!)
- 'Now I have to keep it up and hopefully get pregnant one day!'

⇨ JESSICA'S STORY

'I first suspected something was up when I came off the Pill last summer. I'd never really suffered from acne before, just the occasional spot. Nor had my periods ever really been too irregular – they were never exactly like clockwork, but when I came off the Pill I'd skip them altogether one month and then get them between three and nine weeks later. There was no knowing when and if it would come. So I went to the doctor.

'One blood test later, my GP told me I was suffering from PCOS. I knew what it was – one of my closest friends was diagnosed a couple of years ago. It was a shock to the system, especially when my GP told me there was nothing I could do about it (though she did arrange for me to go for an ultrasound). She then proceeded to tell me the only time PCOS would be a problem for me was when I wanted to conceive. I was shocked and speechless. Nothing was given to me – no leaflets, no information about further reading or support groups.

'So I took my health into my own hands. After reading on the internet and buying a copy of *The PCOS Diet Book* (which I can't recommend enough!), I changed my diet. Not radically – I'd always been pretty healthy, but swapped white flour for wholemeal and made sure I ate more fruit and vegetables, and – as far as budget and availability would allow – went organic. I also snacked on nuts and dried fruit instead of crisps and chocolate, or the other extreme of starving myself! And after 28 years of barely no exercise, I went on a 10-minute jog every other day, which I quickly came to love and, to my complete surprise, look forward to!

'Eight weeks after the GP's diagnosis I'd definitely lost weight and my spots were clearing up. But still no period. This upset me dreadfully. I felt despair. I'd never be able to have a baby. I was a freak, not quite a 100 per cent woman. Another week passed. Still no period. So on the off-chance I bought a pregnancy test one evening on the way home from work. As soon as I got in I went to the loo and did the test, without saying a word about it to my partner (over the months leading up to the PCOS diagnosis I'd thought I could be pregnant so many times I felt a bit like the boy who cried wolf). To my utmost surprise, the test was positive. I was pregnant.'

⇨ SAM'S STORY

'At this moment I am listening to my 3-month-old son scream his little lungs out. I didn't ever think I would enjoy that sound so much.

'I was diagnosed with PCOS in 2001, and after a miscarriage I switched doctors. The doctor actually listened to me and set me up on a healthy diet and exercise routine and a prescription for metformin. Within two months I had lost 16 lb, and was pregnant in another four months. For all of you out there, don't give up. Be persistent. If your doctor isn't listening to you, find one who will. Do your research about the different treatments and know your info. I am going back to the Vitex now that I am postpartum and am going to eat healthily for the rest of my life.'

⇨ JILL'S STORY

'I was diagnosed with PCOS two years after stopping birth control pills. On the Pill I'd gained 40 lb, which I believe started insulin resistance in my body. I had no periods at all for two years. The doctors wanted to put me back on birth control pills to "fix" the problem. I refused.

'I started doing research on the Internet. After much prayer and guidance, I supplemented my diet with a multivitamin, trace minerals, magnesium, chromium, vitamin E and flaxseed oil. I also changed my diet. I ate nothing with white flour as an ingredient. I stopped eating meat since it slows digestion. I added salads and fruits to my staples.

'I implemented an exercise routine of three times a week for 30–45 minutes of walking or riding my bike. It took a year to implement all these things, and I thought sometimes that I was going too far, that maybe I was over-reacting, but I just had to follow the cues of my body.

'Well, after having a period for three months, my husband and I conceived. I am 25 weeks' pregnant with a baby girl. This is truly a miracle and worth all the years of trying to learn how my body ticks. I hope everyone going through this can find a treatment and approach that works best for them.'

⇨ REBECCA'S STORY

'My daughter of 17 was diagnosed nine months ago with PCOS. I have PCOS too and this was the trigger I needed to sort myself out.

'I put my daughter and myself on a new healthy eating regime. We drink loads of water, eat stacks of vegetables and fruit, no processed foods, all natural and fresh nuts, seeds and lean meat. When I started this diet with her, I felt a distinct difference in my whole body. I had more energy. I could move more easily, I wanted to stay active. I also lost several pounds.

'I do believe that since we switched to everything natural and organic, or just even fresh and nothing processed, both of us are healthier. My daughter is dating for the first time. She's glowing with health and a sense of fun. As for me, my PCOS is totally under control and I don't have cramps when I have my periods any more – I also have endometriosis and my cramps in the past have been debilitating; I wouldn't be able to move. Now I don't have that problem. I am now a firm believer in not using products with pesticides on them or processed with other chemicals. It has made a difference in my lifestyle and my overall physical health. I still have more weight to lose, but I know that will come in time.'

⇨ JO'S STORY

'In my early twenties I was diagnosed with PCOS and was told that I wouldn't be able to have children as I only had a period every six to eight months and didn't ovulate. When I was 23 I had an early miscarriage, after that me and my husband tried for a baby. In January 2003 I started having reflexology, as I had heard this was very good for hormonal problems. I had a period a month and a half later, which was a real result for me. In the April I started taking metformin as well as having the reflexology treatments and by the end of that month I was pregnant.

'Three years on I now have a beautiful little girl called Amy-Jane. I also have been having regular monthly periods ever since. I was so pleased with my reflexology treatments that I have now given up my career as an IT specialist and I am now a fully qualified holistic therapist. I now get to help people who were in my position, which is very rewarding.'

▷ **THERESA'S STORY**

'I used to be an energetic person, but everything changed a few months after I stopped taking the Pill. I felt as if I were falling apart. I became anxious and moody; it was difficult to concentrate. I was depressed one moment, agitated the next, perpetually tired. Some days even walking up the stairs was exhausting. I wasn't menstruating and my skin was breaking out in spots and blemishes. My hair lacked shine.

'My doctor referred me to a specialist for a series of tests. I was told that I had polycystic ovaries and that as long as I had this condition it could be hard for me to get pregnant. I was told that the condition was very common. I suppose this was meant to make me feel better, but it didn't really. I heard the word "cyst" and imagined the worst. All I thought was: if the condition is so common why haven't I heard of it? Does this mean I can't have babies?

'Despite feeling anxious it was a huge relief to finally find out what was wrong and to be taken seriously. Without really knowing what was going on, I agreed to have progesterone to encourage a bleed, the fertility drug clomid to induce ovulation, and hormone injections to release the egg if it was ready. It was an emotional roller-coaster of a month when each day seemed the longest ever. The treatment was all I could think about. It was painful and difficult. It wasn't easy for my husband either. I shall never forget the look on his face when I'd had my injection and it was suggested that we have intercourse that evening, the following morning, afternoon and evening, and then again the day after. No pressure on the poor guy, then!

'I jumped for joy when the pregnancy test turned positive after my first attempt. Nine months later I gave birth to a beautiful baby boy, and with the same treatment a year later I had a beautiful baby girl. Now that my family was complete, I really turned my attention to my PCOS. A year after my second baby I still wasn't menstruating. I visited three more doctors and all of them suggested the Pill, but this wasn't what I wanted. I wanted a natural approach. I did lots of my own research and talked to experts, and even wrote a series of articles and a book about hormonal imbalance in women. Then I had a stroke of luck. My editor suggested that I get together with fellow PCOS sufferer, Colette Harris, who had already written a groundbreaking and bestselling book on the subject of PCOS in women. Colette needed a writer to work with her on *The PCOS Diet Book*, a book designed to encourage women with PCOS to treat their condition through diet, supplements, exercise and stress relief. This was almost too good to be true. I could write, learn about and treat my condition at the same time.

'Over a five-year period the natural approach Colette advocates has worked brilliantly. My periods have returned naturally and have been as regular as clockwork ever since. I've also got my weight under control and my skin and hair look healthy again. Unless we decide to try for another baby I have no way of knowing if my DIY techniques would have resulted in pregnancy, but I do know that I have never felt healthier or happier.'

⇨ COLETTE'S STORY

'I was diagnosed with PCOS in December 1996 after months of failing health (painful acne, hairs sprouting all over the place, piling on the weight, turning into Jekyll and Hyde with awful mood swings) and repeat, repeat, repeat visits to the doctor. At my scan, aged 23, I was told by the technician that I had PCOS but I shouldn't worry, as there was now so much medical help on offer for women who can't have kids. I had no ideas what PCOS was – and neither, really, did my GP, who at least admitted as much and put me on the waiting list to see a specialist X months away.

'So I decided to turn PCOS detective and experiment with some DIY remedies while I waited – something I wouldn't recommend, but I was so desperate, and angry, and able through my work as a health journalist to do by calling every expert and practitioner I knew for advice and trailing through reams of medical papers on the Internet. I changed my diet to the one recommended in this book, started taking *Agnus castus*, EFAs and aromatherapy baths, and my symptoms really did start to recede – weight dropped off me, my spots faded, my hair stopped falling out and my moods evened out. So much so that when I did finally get to see the specialist she asked me to send her information on what I was doing – "it seems to be working better than what I could offer you," was what she said.

'And when she said that, I thought, hang on a minute, maybe other women with PCOS would be interested, too – at that time there were only small support groups, no websites and no books for patients. And that's how I got writing. Ten years later my periods are still regular as clockwork – but the thing I find sabotages them occasionally – and brings back my spots and mood swings to boot – is stress. Not only because of the cortisol and insulin connection, but also because it stops me making the effort to eat as well or finding time to exercise. So that's my resolution for 2006 – curb the stress and put exercise first. I hate to admit it but I always feel 10 times better afterwards!'

If you have a positive story to tell please do it on the chatrooms, websites, in the Verity Newsletter and at support group meetings – it's always great for people to hear the good news about PCOS, not just the bad!

REFERENCES

INTRODUCTION: TAKING CONTROL

1. Kitzinger, C. *et al.*, 'The Thief of Womanhood: Woman's Experience of Polycystic Ovarian syndrome', *Soc Sci Med*, 2002, 54 (3): 349–61
2. Hahn, S. *et al.*, 'Clinical and psychological correlates of quality-of-life in polycystic ovary syndrome', *Eur J Endocrinol.* 2005 Dec; 153 (6): 853–60

PART ONE: THE LOW-DOWN ON PCOS
CHAPTER 1: WHAT EXACTLY IS PCOS?

1. Hart, C. *et al.*, 'Definitions, prevalence and symptoms of polycystic ovaries and polycystic ovary syndrome', *Best Pract Res Clin Obstet Gynaecol.* 2004 Oct; 18 (5): 671–83

2. Hill, K. *et al.*, 'The pathogenesis and treatment of PCOS', *Nurse Pract.* 2003 Jul; 28 (7 Pt 1): 8–17, 22–3, table of contents; quiz 23–5

3. Costello, M. *et al.*, 'Polycystic ovary syndrome – a management update', *Aust Fam Physician.* 2005 Mar; 34 (3): 127–33

4. Sheehan, M. *et al.*, 'Polycystic Ovarian Syndrome: Diagnosis and Management', *Clin Med Res.* 2004 Feb; 2 (1): 13–27

5. Gambineri, R. *et al.*, 'Obesity and the polycystic ovary syndrome', *Int J Obes Relat Metab Disord.* 2002 Jul; 26 (7): 883–96

6. Batt, C. *et al.*, 'Ultrasound evaluation of PCO, PCOS and OHSS', *Reprod Biomed Online.* 2004 Dec; 9 (6): 614–9

7. Cussons, A. *et al.*, 'Polycystic ovarian syndrome: marked differences between endocrinologists and gynaecologists in diagnosis and management', *Clin Endocrinol (Oxf).* 2005 Mar; 62 (3): 289–95. Azziz, R. *et al.*, 'Diagnostic criteria for polycystic ovary syndrome: a reappraisal', *Fertil Steril.* 2005 May; 83 (5): 1343–6. Homburg, R. *et al.*, 'What is polycystic ovarian syndrome? A proposal for a consensus on the definition and diagnosis of polycystic ovarian syndrome', *Hum Reprod.* 2002 Oct; 17 (10): 2495–9

8. Fran, E. *et al.*, 'Genetics of polycystic ovarian syndrome', *Reprod Biomed Online.* 2005 Jun; 10 (6): 713–20

9. Ng, E. *et al.*, 'Are there differences in ultrasound parameters between Chinese women with polycystic ovaries only and with polycystic ovary syndrome?', *Eur J Obstet Gynecol Reprod Biol.* 2005 Sep 1

CHAPTER 2: WHAT CAUSES PCOS?

1. Fratantonio, E. *et al.*, 'Genetics of polycystic ovarian syndrome', *Reprod Biomed Online.* 2005 Jun; 10 (6): 713–20

2. Duskova, M. *et al.*, 'What may be the markers of the male equivalent of polycystic ovary syndrome?', *Physiol Res.* 2004; 53 (3): 287–94

3. Franks, S. *et al.*, 'The genetic basis of polycystic ovary syndrome', *Hum Reprod.* 1997 Dec; 12 (12): 2641–8

4. Waterworth, D. *et al.*, 'Linkage and association of insulin gene VNTR regulatory polymorphism with PCOS', *Lancet* 1997, 349: 1771–2

5. Frantantonio, E. Section of Andrology and Internal Medicine, Department of Biomedical Sciences, University of Catania, Catania, Italy

6. Kumar, A. *et al.*, 'Prevalence of adrenal androgen excess in patients with the polycystic ovary syndrome (PCOS)', *Clin Endocrinol (Oxf).* 2005 Jun; 62 (6): 644–9

7. Grana, M. *et al.*, 'Subcutaneous administration of pulsatile gonadotropin-releasing hormone decreases serum follicle-stimulating hormone and luteinizing hormone levels in women with polycystic ovary syndrome: a preliminary study', *Fertil Steril.* 2005 May; 83 (5): 1466–72

8. Ardawi, M. *et al.*, 'Plasma adiponectin and insulin resistance in women with polycystic ovary syndrome', *Fertil Steril.* 2005 Jun; 83 (6): 1708–16

9. Prelevic, G. *et al.*, 'Insulin resistance in polycystic ovary syndrome', *Curr Opin Obstet Gynecol.* 1997 Jun; 9 (3): 193–201

10. Panidis, D. *et al.*, 'Serum parathyroid hormone concentrations are increased in women with polycystic ovary syndrome', *Clin Chem.* 2005 Sep; 51 (9): 1691–7. Epub 2005 Jul 21

11. Pallotti, S. *et al.*, 'Relationship between insulin secretion, and thyroid and ovary function in patients suffering from polycystic ovary', *Minerva Endocrinol.* 2005 Sep; 30 (3): 193–7

12. Gallinelli, I. *et al.*, 'Autonomic and neuroendocrine responses to stress in patients with functional hypothalamic secondary amenorrhea', *Fertil Steril.* 2000, Apr 73 (4) 812–6

13. Dr Mark Leondires, Medical Director and lead physician, Reproductive Medicine Associates of Connecticut (RMA-CT) Norwalk, USA

14. Dumesic, D. *et al.*, 'Early origins of polycystic ovary syndrome', *Reprod Fertil Dev.* 2005; 17 (3): 349–60

15. Cresswell, J. *et al.*, 'Fetal growth, length of gestation, and polycystic ovaries in adult life', *Lancet* 1997 Oct 18; 350 (9085): 1131–5

16. Clark, A. *et al.*, 'Weight loss results in significant improvement in pregnancy and ovulation rates in annovulatory obese women', *Human Reproduction* 10 (1995) 2705–12. Kiddy, D. *et al.*, 'Improvement in endocrine and ovarian function during dietary treatment of obese women with PCOS', *Clin Endocrin* 36 (1992) 105–11

17. Sindelka, G. *et al.*, 'Can hormonal contraceptives affect plasma levels of IGF-1 and IGFBP-1 in slim women with polycystic ovary syndrome?', *Cas Lek Cesk.* 2001 Aug 2; 140 (15): 469–72

18. McCluskey, S. *et al.*, 'Polycystic ovary syndrome and bulimia', *Fertil Steril.* 1991 Feb; 55 (2): 287–91

19. Pasquali, R. *et al.*, 'Role of changes in dietary habits in polycystic ovary syndrome', *Reprod Biomed Online.* 2004 Apr; 8 (4): 431–9

20. Dr Samuel Thatcher, Reproductive Expert and author of *PCOS: The Hidden Epidemic* (Perspectives Press)

21. Tsutsumi, O. *et al.*, 'Assessment of human contamination of estrogenic endocrine-disrupting chemicals and their risk for human reproduction', *J Steroid Biochem Mol Biol.* 2005 Feb; 93 (2–5): 325–30. Epub 2005 Jan 26

22. Harden, C. *et al.*, 'Polycystic ovaries and polycystic ovary syndrome in epilepsy: evidence for neurogonadal disease', *Epilepsy Curr.* 2005 Jul–Aug; 5 (4): 142–6

23. Weiner, C. *et al.*, 'Androgens and mood dysfunction in women: comparison of women with polycystic ovarian syndrome to healthy controls', *Psychosom Med.* 2004 May–Jun; 66 (3): 356–62

24. Goodarzi, M. *et al.*, 'Beta-Cell function: a key pathological determinant in polycystic ovary syndrome', *J Clin Endocrinol Metab.* 2005 Jan; 90 (1): 310–5. Epub 2004 Oct 26

25. Dokras, A. *et al.*, 'Screening women with polycystic ovary syndrome for metabolic syndrome', *Obstet Gynecol.* 2005 Jul; 106 (1): 131–7

CHAPTER 3: PCOS AND YOUR LIFE STAGES – FROM PUBERTY TO MENOPAUSE

1. Buggs, C. *et al.*, 'Polycystic ovary syndrome in adolescence', *Endocrinol Metab Clin North Am.* 2005 Sep; 34 (3): 677–705

2. Kakani, K. *et al.*, 'Polycystic ovary syndrome, diabetes and cardiovascular disease: risks and risk factors', *J Obstet Gynaecol.* 2004 Sep; 24 (6): 613–21

3. Fujiwara, K. *et al.*, 'Skipping breakfast is associated with dysmenorrhea in young women in Japan', *Int J Food Sci Nutr.* 2003 Nov; 54 (6): 505–9

4. Ibanez, L. *et al.*, 'Polycystic ovary syndrome after precocious pubarche: ontogeny of the low-birthweight effect', *Clin Endocrinol (Oxf).* 2001 Nov; 55 (5): 667–72

5. Rai, R. *et al.*, 'Polycystic ovaries and recurrent miscarriage – a reappraisal', *Hum Reprod.* 2000 Mar; 15 (3): 612–5

6. Weer, A. *et al.*, 'Prevalence of gestational diabetes mellitus and pregnancy outcomes in Asian women with polycystic ovary syndrome', *Gynecol Endocrinol.* 2004 Sep; 19 (3): 134–40

7. Kashyap, P. *et al.*, 'Polycystic ovary disease and the risk of pregnancy-induced hypertension', *J Reprod Med.* 2000 Dec; 45 (12): 991–4

8. Margolin, E. *et al.*, 'Polycystic ovary syndrome in post-menopausal women – marker of the metabolic syndrome', *Maturitas.* 2005 Apr 11; 50 (4): 331–6

CHAPTER 4: WHAT AM I DEALING WITH?

1. Hartz, A. *et al.*, 'The association of obesity with infertility and related menstrual abnormalities in women', *Int J Obes.* 1979; 3 (1): 57–73

2. Evans, D. *et al.*, 'Relationship of androgenic activity to body fat topography, fat cell morphology aberrations in premenopausal women', *J Clin Endocrinol Metab.* 57 (1983) 304–10

3. Robinson, S. *et al.*, 'Postprandial thermogenesis is reduced in polycystic ovary syndrome and is associated with increased insulin resistance', *Clin Endocrin* 36 (1992) 537–43

4. Lefe, P. *et al.*, 'Long-term risks of polycystic ovaries syndrome', *Gynecol Obstet Fertil.* 2004 Mar; 32 (3): 193–8

5. Ibid.

6. Balen, A. *et al.*, 'Polycystic ovary syndrome and cancer', *Hum Reprod Update.* 2001 Nov–Dec; 7 (6): 522–5

7. Michelmore, M. *et al.*, 'Polycystic Ovaries and eating disorders: Are they linked?', *Human Reprod* 2001 Apr; 16 (4): 765–9

8. Gallinelli, I. *et al.*, 'Autonomic and neuroendocrine responses to stress in patients with functional hypothalamic secondary amenorrhea', *Fertil Steril.* 2000 Apr; 73 (4): 812–6

9. 'Sex hormones as risk factor? More asthma in cases of irregular menstrual periods', *MMW Fortschr Med.* 2002 Oct 31; 144 (44): 14

CHAPTER 5: HOW CAN MY DOCTOR HELP?

1. British Medical Association, *Official Guide to Medicines and Drugs* (Dorling Kindersley, 1998): 147

2. University of Southern California School of Medicine research study, 'Mini pill increases risk of Diabetes', *Journal of the American Medical Association*, Aug 12, 1998

3. Baillargeon, J.P. *et al.*, 'Association between the current use of low-dose oral contraceptives and cardiovascular arterial disease: a meta-analysis', *J Clin Endocrinol Metab.* 2005 Jul; 90 (7): 3863–70

4. 'Nutrition and the pill', *Journal of rep Med* 29 (7) July 1984, Suppl 547–50

5. University of Southern California School of Medicine research study, 'Mini pill increases risk of Diabetes,' *Journal of the American Medical Association*, Aug 12, 1998

6. Clayton, W.J. *et al.*, 'A randomized controlled trial of laser treatment among hirsute women with polycystic ovary syndrome', *Br J Dermatol.* 2005 May; 152 (5): 986–92

7. La Marcia *et al.*, 'Metformin treatment of PCOS during adolescence and the reproductive period', *Eur J Obstet Gynecol Reprod Biol.* 2005 Jul 1; 121 (1): 3–7

8. Harborne, L. *et al.*, 'Metformin and weight loss in obese women with polycystic ovary syndrome: comparison of doses', *J Clin Endocrinol Metab.* 2005 Aug; 90 (8): 4593–8. Epub 2005 May 10

9. Qublan, H. *et al.*, 'Metformin in the treatment of clomiphene citrate-resistant women with high BMI and primary infertility: clinical results and reproductive outcome', *J Obstet Gynaecol.* 2005 Jan; 25 (1): 55–9. Heard, M.J. *et al.*, 'Pregnancies following use of metformin for ovulation induction in patients with polycystic ovary syndrome', *Fertil Steril*, 2002, 77 (4): 669–73. A study of 48 women with PCOS and infertility was conducted at the Baylor College of Medicine. They were first given metformin and 19 of them resumed menstruating and showed indications of ovulation. But 10 required clomiphene (a fertility drug) in addition to metformin in order to show evidence of ovulation. Twenty women of the 48 (42 per cent) became pregnant. However, 7 of the 20 miscarried.

10. Jakubowicz, D.J. *et al.*, 'Effects of metformin on early pregnancy loss in the polycystic ovary syndrome', *J Clin Endocrinol Metab*, 2002, 87 (2): 524–9. Research from the Hospital de Clinicas Caracas in Venezuela looked at 65 women who received Glucophage during their pregnancies versus 31 who did not. The early pregnancy (first trimester) loss rate in the metformin group was 8.8 per cent as compared to a 41.9 per cent loss in the untreated group.

11. Brock, B. *et al.*, 'Is metformin therapy for polycystic ovary syndrome safe during pregnancy?' *Basic Clin Pharmacol Toxicol.* 2005 Jun; 96 (6): 410–2

12. 'Effects of inositol on ovarian function and metabolic factors in women with PCOS: a randomized double blind placebo-controlled trial', *Eur Rev Med Pharmacol Sci.* 2003 Nov–Dec; 7 (6): 151–9

13. Norman, R. *et al.*, 'The role of lifestyle modification in polycystic ovary syndrome', *Trends Endocrinol Metab.* 2002 Aug; 13 (6): 251–7

PART TWO: TOTAL TLC FOR YOUR BODY: ACTION PLAN FOR YOUR HEALTH NOW AND IN THE FUTURE

CHAPTER 6: YOUR PCOS NUTRITION GUIDE

1. Marsh, K. *et al.*, 'The optimal diet for women with polycystic ovary syndrome?', *Br J Nutr.* 2005 Aug; 94 (2): 154–65. Tolino, A. *et al.*, 'Evaluation of ovarian functionality after a dietary treatment in obese women with polycystic ovary syndrome', *Eur J Obstet Gynecol Reprod Biol.* 2005 Mar 1; 119 (1): 87–93. Pasquali, A. *et al.*, 'Role of changes in dietary habits in polycystic ovary syndrome', *Reprod Biomed Online.* 2004 Apr; 8 (4): 431–9

2. Al, M. *et al.*, 'The effect of obesity on the outcome of infertility management in women with polycystic ovary syndrome', *Arch Gynecol Obstet.* 2004 Dec; 270 (4): 205–10. Epub 2003 Aug 29. Tolstoi, L. *et al.*, 'Weight Loss and Medication in Polycystic Ovary Syndrome Therapy', *Nutr Today.* 2002 Mar; 37 (2): 57–62

3. From issue 2526 of *New Scientist* magazine, 17 November 2005, page 12

4. Brand, Miller J. *et al.*, 'The optimal diet for women with polycystic ovary syndrome?', *Br J Nutr.* 2005 Aug; 94 (2): 154–65

5. Gerber, M. *et al.*, 'Fibre and breast cancer', *Eur J cancr Prev* 1998 May; 7 suppl 2; S63–7

6. Bjork, I. *et al.*, 'The glycaemic index: importance of dietary fibre and other food properties', *Proc Nutr Soc.* 2003 Feb; 62 (1): 201–6

7. Lau, K. *et al.*, 'Synergistic Interactions Between Commonly Used Food Additives in a Developmental Neurotoxicity Test', *Toxicol Sci.* 2005 Dec 13

8. Chan, J. *et al.*, 'Water, other fluids and fatal coronary heart disease,' *Am J Epidemiol* 2002 Jan 155 (9): 827–33

9. Willett, W. *et al.*, 'Intake of trans fatty acids and risk of coronary heart disease among women', *Lancet* 1993 Mar 6; 341 (8845):581–5

10. Kasim, K. *et al.*, 'Metabolic and endocrine effects of a polyunsaturated fatty acid-rich diet in polycystic ovary syndrome', *J Clin Endocrinol Metab.* 2004 Feb; 89 (2): 615–20

11. Lefevre, M. *et al.*, 'Dietary fatty acids, hemostasis, and cardiovascular disease risk', *J Am Diet Assoc.* 2004 Mar; 104 (3): 410–9; quiz 492. Saldeen, P. *et al.*, 'Women and omega-3 Fatty acids', *Obstet Gynecol Surv.* 2004 Oct; 59 (10): 722–30; quiz 745–6. Review

12. Researchers from the University of Navarra followed the dairy consumption of 6,000 people for a two-year period between 2003 and 2005. They found that those who drank skimmed milk and took other dairy products, but not full-fat milk, were 50 per cent less likely to suffer from high blood pressure compared to those who consumed little or no skimmed milk and dairy products.

13. Sab, T. *et al.*, 'Oxidative stress in polycystic ovary syndrome and its contribution to the risk of cardiovascular disease', *Clin Biochem.* 2001 Jul; 34 (5): 407–13. Fenkci, I. *et al.*, 'Decreased total antioxidant status and increased oxidative stress in women with polycystic ovary syndrome may contribute to the risk of cardiovascular disease', *Fertil Steril.* 2003 Jul; 80 (1): 123–7

14. Barnes, S. *et al.*, 'Soy isoflavones – phytoestrogens and what else?', *J Nutr.* 2004 May; 134 (5): 1225S–1228S

15. Stark, A. *et al.*, 'Phytoestrogens: a review of recent findings', *J Pediatr Endocrinol Metab.* 2002 May; 15 (5): 561–72

16. Keck, A. *et al.*, 'Cruciferous vegetables: cancer protective mechanisms of glucosinolate hydrolysis products and selenium', *Integr Cancer Ther.* 2004 Mar; 3 (1): 5–12. Review

CHAPTER 7: EXERCISE –YOUR PCOS-BEATING PLAN

1. Huber-Buchholz, M.M. *et al.*, 'Restoration of reproductive potential by lifestyle modification in obese polycystic ovary syndrome: role of insulin sensitivity and luteinizing hormone', *J Clin Endocrinol Metab.* 1999 Apr; 84 (4): 1470–4

2. Giannopoulou, I. *et al.*, 'Exercise is required for visceral fat loss in postmenopausal women with type 2 diabetes', *J Clin Endocrinol Metab.* Dec 14, 2004

3. Randeva, H.S. *et al.*, 'Exercise decreases plasma total homocysteine in overweight young women with polycystic ovary syndrome', *J Clin Endocrinol Metab.* 2002; 87 (10): 4496–501

4. According to a study published in the October 2005 *Journal of Applied Psychology* even moderate exercise can 'put the brakes on' the accumulation of waist fat, women with PCOS are prone to. Researchers at Duke University Centre in South Carolina found that the quality of exercise was more important than the amount. Lead researcher Dr Cris Slentz said that people who were already overweight could significantly decrease abdominal fat and increase their health levels by doing the most low-intensity forms of exercise,

such as cycling on a stationary bike or walking on a treadmill. The team found that those who worked out moderately for about three hours each week did as well as those who did high-intensity exercise for two hours a week. Both groups showed no significant gain in deep abdominal fat, while their sedentary peers saw an abdominal fat gain of almost 10 per cent over six months.

5. McAuley, K. *et al.*, 'Intensive lifestyle changes are necessary to improve insulin sensitivity: A randomized controlled trial', *Diabetes Care* 2002 Mar; 25 (3): 445–52

6. 'Fatigue; Feeling tired too much of the time', *Harvard Health Letter* 22 (10): 1–3, Aug 1997

CHAPTER 8: YOUR HEALTH-BOOSTING LIFESTYLE DETOX

1. Friends of the Earth Press Briefing for safer chemicals campaign: Chemicals and Health http://www.foe.co.uk/campaigns/safer_chemicals/issues/health_threats/index.html

2. Sirakov, M. *et al.*, 'Xenoestrogens – danger for the future generations?' *Akush Ginekol (Sofiia)* 2004; 43 (4): 39–45

3. Singleton, D. *et al.*, 'Xenoestrogen exposure and mechanisms of endocrine disruption', *Front Biosci* 2003 Jan 1; 8: s110–8

4. http://news.bbc.co.uk/1/hi/uk/1877162.stm

5. Xang, X. *et al.*, 'Intake of trans fatty acids and risk of coronary heart disease among women', *Lancet* 1993 Mar 6; 341 (8845): 581–5

6. Norman, J. *et al.*, 'The role of lifestyle modification in polycystic ovary syndrome', *Trends Endocrinol Metab.* 2002 Aug; 13 (6): 251–7

7. Johnston, K. *et al.*, 'Coffee acutely modifies gastrointestinal hormone secretion and glucose tolerance in humans: glycemic effects of chlorogenic acid and caffeine', *Am J Clin Nutr* 2003 Oct; 78 (4): 728–33

8. Curtis, J. *et al.*, 'Effects of cigarette smoking, caffeine consumption, and alcohol intake on fecundability', *Am J Epidemiol* 1997 Jul 1; 146 (1): 32–41

9. Agardh, E. *et al.*, 'Coffee consumption, type 2 diabetes and impaired glucose tolerance in Swedish men and women', *J Intern Med.* 2004 Jun; 255 (6): 645–52

10. 'Endocrine Disruption Induced by Organochlorines (OCs): Field Studies And Experimental Models', *J Toxicol Environ Health A* 2006 Jan; 69 (1): 53–76. 'Possible health impact of phytoestrogens and xenoestrogens in food', *APMIS* 2001 Mar; 109 (3): 161–84

11. Nuti, F. *et al.*, 'Synthesis of DEHP metabolites as biomarkers for GC-MS evaluation of phthalates as endocrine disrupters', *Bioorg Med Chem* 2005 May 16; 13 (10): 3461–5

12. Kroenke, C. *et al.*, 'A cross-sectional study of alcohol consumption patterns and biologic markers of glycemic control among 459 women', *Diabetes Care* 2003 Jul; 26 (7): 1971–8

13. http://news.bbc.co.uk/1/hi/health/3545684.stm/ http://www.dwi.gov.uk/pressrel/2004/pr0304.shtm

14. An article published in the *Journal of Applied Toxology* has claimed that using underarm deodorant may increase the risk of breast cancer. Dr Darbre said that the aluminium compounds used in deodorants to block sweat glands could pass through the skin, possibly aided by cuts as a result of shaving, and then mimic the oestrogen hormone. Deodorant manufacturers have reassured customers that their products are safe as other experts and charities stressed that no proof for this assertion has yet been offered.

CHAPTER 9: THE BEST NUTRITIONAL AND HERBAL SUPPLEMENTS

1. 'Insulin resistance: lifestyle and nutritional interventions', *Altern Med Rev.* 2000 Apr; 5 (2): 109–32

2. 'A scientific review: the role of chromium in insulin resistance', *Diabetes Educ* 2004; Suppl: 2–14

3. Preuss, H. *et al.*, 'Effects of a natural extract of (-)-hydroxycitric acid (HCA-SX) and a combination of HCA-SX plus niacin-bound chromium and Gymnema sylvestre extract on weight loss', *Diabetes Obes Metab* 2004 May; 6 (3): 171–80

4. 'A scientific review: the role of chromium in insulin resistance', *Diabetes Educ* 2004; Suppl: 2–14

5. Kidd, S. *et al.*, 'The effects of pyridoxine on pituitary hormone secretion in amenorrhea-galactorrhea syndromes', *J Clin Endocrinol Metab* 1982 Apr; 54 (4): 872–5

6. Thys-Jacobs, S., *et al.*, 'Vitamin D and calcium dysregulation in the polycystic ovarian syndrome', *Steroids* 1999 Jun; 64 (6): 430–5

7. Mathieu, C. *et al.*, 'Vitamin D and diabetes', *Diabetologia* 2005 Jul; 48 (7): 1247–57. Epub 2005 Jun 22

8. Harkness, E. *et al.*, 'Calcium and vitamin D status in the adolescent: key roles for bone, body weight, glucose tolerance, and estrogen biosynthesis', *J Pediatr Adolesc Gynecol.* 2005 Oct; 18 (5): 305–11

9. Ilich, J. *et al.*, 'A lighter side of calcium: role of calcium and dairy foods in body weight', *Arh Hig Rada Toksikol.* 2005 Mar; 56 (1): 33–8

10. Yokota, K. *et al.*, 'Diabetes mellitus and magnesium', *Clin Calcium* 2005 Feb; 15 (2): 203–12

11. Ebbesson, O. *et al.*, 'Omega-3 fatty acids improve glucose tolerance and components of the metabolic syndrome in Alaskan Eskimos: the Alaska Siberia project', *Int J Circumpolar Health* 2005 Sep; 64 (4): 396–408

12. Singh, R.B. *et al.*, 'Effect of hydrosoluble coenzyme Q10 on blood pressures and insulin resistance in hypertensive patients with coronary artery disease', *J Hum Hypertens.* 1999; 13 (3): 203–208. Kelly, G. *et al.*, 'Insulin resistance: lifestyle and nutritional interventions', *Altern Med Rev.* 2000 Apr; 5 (2): 109–32

13. Nestler, J.E. *et al.*, 'Ovulatory and metabolic effects of D-chiro-inositol in the polycystic ovary syndrome', *Engl J Med.* 1999 Apr 29; 340 (17): 1314–20. Iuorno, M.J. *et al.*, 'Effects of d-chiro-inositol in lean women with the polycystic ovary syndrome', *Endocr Pract.* 2002 Nov–Dec; 8 (6): 417–23

14. Gerli, S. *et al.*, 'Effects of inositol on ovarian function and metabolic factors in women with PCOS: a randomized double blind placebo-controlled trial', *Eur Rev Med Pharmacol Sci.* 2003 Nov–Dec; 7 (6): 151–9

15. A chasteberry preparation was given to 3,162 women to assess the effectiveness of vitex for corpus luteum insufficiency. Some 77.4 per cent had menstrual cycle disturbances of various types, and the others suffered from a range of gynaecological problems. The average length of treatment was 5 months. The women reported rated the results as completely effective (33 per cent), significantly improved (55 per cent), and no change (7 per cent). Their doctors reported very good results in 68 per cent of cases, adequate in 22 per cent, and no change in 7 per cent. Loch, E.G., 'Gynaecology in practice – A sure choice of therapy', *Tjherapiewoche* 1993, 43 (48): 2577–80

16. Twenty women with secondary amenorrhoea took a chasteberry extract for 6 months. Lab testing was done to measure progesterone, FSH and LH, and pap smears were done at the beginning of the study, at 3 months, and at 6 months. At the end of the study, the researchers were able to evaluate 15 of the women. Ten out of the 15 women had a return of their menstrual cycles. Testing showed that values for progesterone and LH increased, and FSH values either didn't change or decreased slightly. Loch, E. *et al.*, 'Diagnosis and treatment of dyshormonal menstrual periods in the general practice', *Gynakol Praxis* 1990, 14 (3): 489–95

17. Eighteen women with abnormally low progesterone levels were given vitex daily. After 3 months of treatment, 13 showed increases in progesterone, and 2 became pregnant. Propping, D. *et al.*, 'Treatment of corpus luteum insufficiency', *Zeitscchrift Fur Allgemein* 1987, 63: 932–3

18. Fifty-two women with luteal phase defects due to latent hyperprolactinemia (high prolactin levels) were given either vitex or a placebo. Prolactin levels were normalized after 3 months in the treatment group, and deficits in luteal progesterone production were eliminated. Two of the women became pregnant. Milewicz, A., *et al.*, 'Vitex agnus castus extract in the treatment of luteal phase defects due to latent hyperprolactinaemia. Results of a randomized placebo-controlled double-blind study', *Arzniem-Forschung* 1993, 43 (II–7): 752–6

19. Thirteen women with high prolactin levels and irregular cycles were given a vitex compound. Their prolactin levels fell, and normal menstrual cycles returned to all of the women. Bleier, V. W., 'Therapie von zyklus-und blutungsstrorungen und weiteren endokrin bedingten erkrankungen der frau mit pflanzlichen wirkstoffen', *Zbl Gynakologie* 1959, 18: 701–9

20. A chasteberry preparation was used in women with menstrual cycle abnormalities. Acne was either eliminated or improved during treatment. In another study, 117 women with four different types of acne were treated with a chasteberry preparation for 1–2 years. Improvement was seen after 6 weeks; by 3 months, about 70 per cent were free of acne. Some treatment relapses were observed after 3–6 weeks. Giss, G. *et al.*, 'Phytotherapeutische behandlung der akne', *Haut- und Gesch* 1968, 43: 645

21. Girman, A. *et al.*, 'An integrative medicine approach to premenstrual syndrome', *Am J Obstet Gynecol.* 2003 May; 188 (5 Suppl): S56–65

22. 'Cinnamon Extract Prevents the Insulin Resistance Induced by a High-fructose Diet', *Horm Metab Res.* 2004 Feb; 36 (2): 119–25. 'Cinnamon Improves Glucose and Lipids of People With Type 2 Diabetes', *Diabetes Care* 2003 Dec; 26 (12): 3215–3218

23. 'Echinacea and the common cold', *Child Health Alert* 2005 Sep; 24: 4

24. Basch, E. *et al.*, 'Therapeutic applications of fenugreek', *Altern Med Rev.* 2003 Feb; 8 (1): 20–7

25. Yeh, G. *et al.*, 'Systematic review of herbs and dietary supplements for glycemic control in diabetes', *Diabetes Care* 2003 Apr; 26 (4): 1277–94

26. Rainone, F. *et al.*, 'Milk thistle', *Am Fam Physician* 2005 Oct 1; 72 (7): 1285–8

27. The team's results were published in the February 2006 issue of *Fertility and Sterility* and this was the first paper to show the association between PCOS and NAFLD

28. Panossian, A. *et al.*, 'Stimulating effect of adaptogens: an overview with particular reference to their efficacy following single dose administration', *Phytother Res.* 2005 Oct; 19 (10): 819–38

29. Sakai, A. *et al.*, 'Induction of Ovulation by Sairei-to for PCOS patients,' *Endocr Clin Nut* 1999, 46; 217–20

30. Netall, T., 'Comparison of Saw Palmetto and Cernitin on prostate growth in rats', *Mol Cell Biochem* 2003 Aug; 250 (1–2) 21–6

31. Russel, L. *et al.*, 'Phytoestrogens, a viable option?' *Am J Med Sci* 2002, Oct; 324 (4) 185–8

32. Ushiroyama, T. *et al.*, 'Effects of unkei-to, an herbal medicine, on endocrine function and ovulation in women with high levels of lutenizing hormone secretion,' *J Reprod Med.* 2001 May; 46 (5) 451–6

CHAPTER 10: HOW NATURAL THERAPIES CAN HELP YOU

1. Shimbo, D. *et al.*, 'Role of depression and inflammation in incident coronary heart disease events', *Am J Cardiol.* 2005 Oct 1; 96 (7): 1016–21

2. Claraco, A.E. *et al.*, 'The reporting of clinical acupuncture research: what do clinicians need to know?' *J Altern Complement Med* 2003 Feb 9 (1) 143–9

3. Stener-Victorin, E. *et al.*, 'Effects of electro-acupuncture on anovulation in women with polycystic ovary syndrome', *Acta Obstet Gynecol Scand.* 2000 Mar; 79 (3): 180–8. Paulus, W.E. *et al.*, 'Influence of acupuncture on the pregnancy rate in patients who undergo assisted reproduction therapy', *Fertility and Sterility* April 2002, 77 (4): 721–724

4. Ernst, E. *et al.*, 'Autogenic training for stress and anxiety: a systematic review', *Complement Ther Med.* 2000 Jun; 8 (2): 106–10. Kanji, N. *et al.*, 'Management of pain through autogenic training', *Complement Ther Nurs Midwifery* 2000 Aug; 6 (3): 143–8

5. 'Research on homeopathy: state of the art', *J Altern Complement Med.* 2005 Oct; 11 (5): 813–29

CHAPTER 11: HOW TO MANAGE YOUR WEIGHT

1. Stad, L. *et al.*, 'Management of infertility in women with polycystic ovary syndrome: a practical guide', *Treat Endocrinol.* 2005; 4 (5): 279–92

2. Gambineri, A. *et al.*, 'Obesity and the polycystic ovary syndrome', *Int J Obes Relat Metab Disord.* 2002 Jul; 26 (7): 883–96. Hartz, A. *et al.*, 'The association of obesity with infertility and related menstrual abnormalities in women', *Int J of Obesity* 3 (1979) 57–73. Saheli, I. *et al.*, 'Pathogenesis of polycystic ovary syndrome: what's the role of obesity?', *Metabolism* 2004 Mar; 53 (3): 358–76. Draveka, I. *et al.*, 'Obesity is the major factor determining an insulin sensitivity and androgen production in women with anovulary cycles', *Bratisl Lek Listy.* 2003; 104 (12): 393–9

3. Wright, C.E. *et al.*, 'Dietary intake, physical activity, and obesity in women with polycystic ovary syndrome', *Int J Obes Relat Metab Discord*, 2004, 28 (8): 1026–32

4. Holte, J. 'Polycystic ovary syndrome and insulin resistance: thrifty genes struggling with over-feeding and sedentary life style?', *J Endocrinol Invest*, 1998, 21 (9): 589–601. San Millan, S. *et al.*, 'Association of the polycystic ovary syndrome with genomic variants related to insulin resistance, type 2 diabetes mellitus, and obesity', *J Clin Endocrinol Metab*, 2004, 89 (6): 2640–6. Friedman, J.M., 'A war on obesity, not the obese', *Science* 2003 Feb 7; 299 (5608): 856–8

5. Ertuck, E. *et al.*, 'Serum leptin levels correlate with obesity parameters but not with hyperinsulinism in women with polycystic ovary syndrome', *Fertil Steril.* 2004 Nov; 82 (5): 1364–8

6. Jequier, E. 'Leptin signaling, adiposity, and energy balance', *Ann NY Acad Sci* 2002, Jun, 967: 379–88. Banks, W.A. *et al.*, 'Triglycerides induce leptin resistance at the blood-brain barrier', *Diabetes* 2004 May; 53 (5): 1253–60

7. Wasko, R. *et al.*, 'Elevated ghrelin plasma levels in patients with polycystic ovary syndrome', *Horm Metab Res.* 2004 Mar; 36 (3): 170–3. Schofl, C., 'Circulating ghrelin levels in patients with polycystic ovary syndrome', *J Clin Endocrinol Metab.* 2002, 87 (10): 4607–10. Moran, L.J. *et al.*, 'Ghrelin and measures of satiety are altered in polycystic ovary syndrome but not differentially affected by diet composition', *J Clin Endocrinol Metab.* 2004, 89 (7): 3337–44

8. Linden-Hirschberg, A.L. *et al.*, 'Impaired cholecystokinin secretion and disturbed appetite regulation in women with polycystic ovary syndrome', *Gynecol Endocrinol.* 2004 Aug; 19 (2): 79–87

9. Robinson, S. *et al.*, 'Postprandial thermogenesis is reduced in PCOS and is associated with increased insulin resistance', *Clin Endor* 36 (1992) 537–43

10. Schwartz, M.W. *et al.*, 'Reduced insulin secretion: an independent predictor of body weight gain', *J Clin Endocrinol Metab.* 1995, 80: 1571–1576

11. Faloia, E. *et al.*, 'Body composition, fat distribution and metabolic characteristics in lean and obese women with polycystic ovary syndrome', *J Endocrinol Invest.* 2004 May; 27 (5): 424–9

12. Evans, G.W. *et al.*, 'Composition and biological activity of chromium-pyridine carbosyalte complexes', *J of Inorganic Biochemistry* 49 (1993): 177–87

13. American Diabetics Association, 'Magnesium Supplementation in the treatment of diabetes', *Diabetes Care* 15 (1992): 1065–7

14. Van Gall, L. *et al.*, 'Biochemical and clinical aspects of co-enzyme Q10', *Journal of Vitaminology* 4 (1984): 369

15. Chasens, E.R. *et al.*, 'Insulin resistance and obstructive sleep apnea: is increased sympathetic stimulation the link?', *Biol Res Nurs.* 2003 Oct; 5 (2): 87–96

16. Fruhbeck, G. *et al.*, 'Obesity: aquaporin enters the picture', *Nature* 2005 Nov 24; 438 (7067): 436–7

CHAPTER 12: FERTILITY-BOOSTING SECRETS THAT WORK

1. Trent, M.E. *et al.*, 'Fertility concerns and sexual behavior in adolescent girls with polycystic ovary syndrome: implications for quality of life', *J Pedatr Adolesc Gynecol.* 2003 Feb 16 (1) 33–7

2. 'Certainly it appears that the risk of miscarriage is increased in mothers with PCOS, as are the risks of gestational diabetes and pregnancy-induced hypertension, unusually small and large babies and c-section rates.' Thatcher, S. *PCOS: The Hidden Epidemic* (Perspectives Press, 2000): 222

3. Homburg, R. *et al.*, 'The management of infertility associated with polycystic ovary syndrome', *Reprod Biol Endocrinol.* 2003 Nov 14: 'In conclusion, there are very few women suffering from anovulatory infertility associated with PCOS who cannot be successfully treated today.'

4. Czeizel, A.E. *et al.*, 'The effect of preconceptional multivitamin supplementation on fertility', *Int J Vitam Nutr Res* 66 (1996): 55–58. Ground-breaking research by the University of Surrey in the UK proves this. The research looked at 367 couples who were trying to conceive

over a period of three years. The women were aged 22 to 45 and the men 25 to 59. Four out of ten had a history of infertility, and the same number had suffered repeated miscarriages. Many, especially those in the older age range, came to the preconception trial as a last resort. Over the past 25 years a British organization called Foresight has pioneered an approach to human fertility that takes into account diet, exposure to pollutants, infections and nutritional status. The couples were instructed to follow a Foresight regime that involves detoxing, being tested for mineral and vitamin deficiencies and having these put right with supplements and by eating organic food. Any infections were treated. By the end of the trial 90 per cent of these couples had given birth to healthy babies. Even 65 per cent of those who had tried IVF without success became pregnant naturally.

5. Marshall, K. *et al.*, 'Polycystic Ovary Syndrome: clinical considerations', *Altern Med Rev.* (2001) Jun 6 (3): 272–92. 'Due to the vast array of side effects associated with many pharmaceutical agents typically prescribed to treat PCOS, natural therapies including nutrient supplementation and botanicals may be a less invasive and equally effective approach.' Richardson, M.R. *et al.*, 'Current perspectives in polycystic ovary syndrome', *Am Fam Physician* 2003 Aug 15; 68 (4): 697–704. Clark, A. *et al.*, 'Weight loss results in significant improvements in pregnancy and ovulation rates in annovulatory obese women', *Human Reproduction* 10 (1995) 2705–12. Kiddy, D. S. *et al.*, 'Improvement in endocrine and ovarian function during dietary treatment of obese women with PCOS', *Clin Endocrin* 36 (1992) 105–11

6. Cikot, R. *et al.*, 'Dutch GPs acknowledge the need for preconceptual health care', *Br J Gen Pract.* (1999) Apr; 49 (441): 314

7. Ontario Early Church Child Development Research Center: 'Preconception and Health; Research and Strategies', *Best Start* brochure 2001

8. Oliva, A. *et al.*, 'Contribution of environmental factors to the risk of male infertility', *Human Reproduction* 16, no. 8 (Aug 2001). Sharpe, R.M. *et al.*, 'Environment, lifestyle and infertility – an intergenerational issue', *Nat Cell Biol.* (2002) Oct; 4 Suppl: s33–40

9. Pasquali, R. *et al.*, 'Obesity and Reproductive disorders in women', *Hum Reprod* update 2003 July–Aug: 9 (4) 360–70. Hertz, A. *et al.*, 'The association of obesity with infertility and related menstrual disorders in women', *International Journal of Obesity* 3 (1979): 57–73. Alieva, E. *et al.*, 'The effect of a decrease in body weight in patients with polycystic ovary syndrome', *Akush Ginekol (mosk)* (1993) 3: 33–6. Clark, A. *et al.*, 'Weight loss results in significant improvements in pregnancy and ovulation rates in annovulatory obese women', *Human Reproduction* 10, 1995. Clark, A. *et al.*, 'Weight loss in obese infertile women results in improvements in reproductive outcome for all forms of fertility treatment', *Human Reprod.* 13, no 6 (1998): 1502ff

10. http://www.newscientist.com/article.ns?id=dn8174

11. Jakobovits, A. *et al.*, 'Interactions of stress and reproduction', *Zentralbl Gynakol.* 2002 Apr; 124 (4): 189–93

12. Domar, A. *et al.*, 'Distress and conception in infertile women: A complementary approach', *Journal of the American MedicalWomen's Association* 45, no 9 (1999)

13. Reiko. K. *et al.*, 'Work-related reproductive disorders among working women', *Industrial Health* (2002) 40 101–112

14. Czeizel, A.E. *et al.*, 'The effect of preconceptional multivitamin supplementation on fertility', *Int JVitam Nutr Res* 66 (1996): 55–58

15. Ward, N. 'Foresight 1990–1993 study of preconceptual care and pregnancy outcome', *J Nutr Environ Med*, 1995, 5: 205–8

16. Gerhard, I. *et al.*, 'Auricular acupuncture in the treatment of female infertility', *Gynaecol Endocrinol* (ENGLAND) Sep 1992, 6 (3): 171

17. Paulus, *et al.*, 'Influence of acupuncture on the pregnancy rate in patients who undergo assisted reproduction therapy', *Fertility and Sterility* 2002, 77 (4)

18. Bergman, J. *et al.*, 'The efficacy of the complex medication Phyto-Hypophyson L in female, hormone-related sterility. A randomized, placebo-controlled clinical double-blind study', *Forsch Komplementarmed Klass Naturheilkd.* 2000 Aug; 7 (4): 190–9

19. Al, T. *et al.*, 'Safety of drugs used in ART', *Drug Saf* 2005; 28 (6): 513–28

20. Domar, A. *et al.*, *Healing Mind, Healthy Woman* (Henry Holt and Co., 1996): 255–57

21. According to new research from the University of Michigan, stress makes a woman three times more likely to miscarry. Nep, P. et al., 'Cortisol levels and early pregnancy loss in humans', *Proc Natl Acad Sci* 2006 Feb 22

CHAPTER 13: FINE-TUNING YOUR TAILOR-MADE PLAN

1. Bijlani, R. *et al.*, 'A brief but comprehensive lifestyle education program based on yoga reduces risk factors for cardiovascular disease and diabetes mellitus', *J Altern Complement Med.* 2005 Apr; 11 (2): 267–74

2. Pallotti, S. *et al.*, 'Relationship between insulin secretion, and thyroid and ovary function in patients suffering from polycystic ovary', *Minerva Endocrinol.* 2005 Sep; 30 (3): 193–7

PART THREE: TAKING CHARGE OF PCOS: NURTURING YOUR EMOTIONS AND SPIRIT

CHAPTER 15: STRESS AND PCOS – HOW TO LET GO AND LIVE BETTER

1. Gallinelli, I. *et al.*, 'Automatic and neuroendocrine responses to stress in patients with functional hypthalmic secondary amenorrhea', *Fertil Steril* 200, April; 73 (4): 812–6

2. Epel, E.S. *et al.*, 'Stress and body shape: stress-induced cortisol secretion is consistently greater among women with central fat', *Psychosom Med* 2000 Sep–Oct; 62 (5): 623–32

3. Epel, E.S. *et al.*, 'Stress may add bite to appetite in women: a laboratory study of stress-induced cortisol and eating behavior', *Psychoneuroendocrinology* 2001 Jan; 26 (1): 37–49

4. Berga, S.L. *et al.*, 'Women with functional hypothalamic amenorrhea but not other forms of anovulation display amplified cortisol concentrations', *Fertil Steril* 1997 Jun; 67 (6): 1024–30. Nepomnaschy, P.A. *et al.*, 'Stress and female reproductive function: a study of daily variations in cortisol, gonadotrophins, and gonadal steroids in the rural Mayan population', *Am J Hum Biol* 2004, 16 (5): 523–32

5. Dole, N. *et al.*, 'Maternal stress and preterm birth', *Am J Epidemiol.* 2003 Jan 1; 157 (1): 14–24. Oths, K.S. *et al.*, 'A prospective study of psychosocial job strain and birth outcomes', *Epidemiology* 2001 Nov; 12 (6): 744–6. Mulder, E.J. *et al.*, 'Prenatal maternal stress: effects on pregnancy and the (unborn) child', *Early Hum Dev* 2002 Dec; 70 (1–2):

3–14. Gallinelli, A. *et al.*, 'Immunological changes and stress are associated with different implantation rates in patients undergoing in vitro fertilization-embryo transfer', *Fert Steril*, 2001, 76 (1): 85–91

6. Berga, S.L. *et al.*, 'The diagnosis and treatment of stress-induced anovulation', *Minerva Ginecol.* 2005, 57 (1): 45–54

7. Tacon, A.M. *et al.*, 'Mindfulness meditation, anxiety reduction, and heart disease: a pilot study', *Fam Community Health* 2003 Jan–Mar; 26 (1): 25–33. Speca, M. *et al.*, 'A randomized, wait-list controlled clinical trial: the effect of a mindfulness meditation-based stress reduction program on mood and symptoms of stress in cancer outpatients', *Psychosom Med.* 2000 Sep–Oct; 62 (5): 613–22

8. Soden, K. *et al.*, 'A randomized controlled trial of aromatherapy massage in a hospice setting', *Palliat Med.* 2004 Mar; 18 (2): 87–92

9. Sianani, G. *et al.*, 'Non-drug therapy in prevention and control of hypertension', *J Assoc Physicians India* 2003 Oct; 51: 1001–6

10. Berga *et al.*, 'Recovery of ovarian activity in women with functional hypothalamic amenorrhea who were treated with cognitive behavior therapy', *Fertility and Sterility* 2003 Oct; 80 (4)

11. Pitkala, L.H. *et al.*, 'Positive life orientation as a predictor of 10-year outcome in an aged population', *J Clin Epidemiol.* 2004 Apr; 57 (4): 409–14

12. Bryant, M.A. *et al.*, 'Sick and tired: does sleep have a vital role in the immune system?', *Nat Rev Immunol.* 2004 Jun; 4 (6): 457–67. Chasens, E.R. *et al.*, 'Insulin resistance and obstructive sleep apnea: is increased sympathetic stimulation the link?', *Biol Res Nurs.* 2003 Oct; 5 (2): 87–96

13. Patel, S.R. 'A prospective study of sleep duration and mortality risk in women', *Sleep* 2004 May 1; 27 (3): 440–4

14. Sanders, M.H. *et al.*, 'Increased risk of obstructive sleep apnea in obese women with polycystic ovary syndrome' (a review of two related articles). Articles reviewed: 'Increased prevalence of obstructive sleep apnea syndrome in obese women with polycystic ovary syndrome' and 'Polycystic ovary syndrome is associated with obstructive sleep apnea and daytime sleepiness: role of insulin resistance', *Sleep Med.* 2002 May; 3 (3): 287–9

CHAPTER 16: COPING WITH DEPRESSION AND LOW MOODS

1. Coffey, S. *et al.*, 'The effect of polycystic ovary syndrome on health-related quality of life', *Gynecol Endocrinol.* 2003 Oct; 17 (5): 379–86. Elsenbruch, S. *et al.*, 'Quality of life, psychosocial well-being, and sexual satisfaction in women with polycystic ovary syndrome', *J Clin Endocrinol Metab.* 2003 Dec; 88 (12): 5801–7. Rasgon, N.L. *et al.*, 'Depression in women with polycystic ovary syndrome: clinical and biochemical correlates', *J Affect Disord.* 2003 May; 74 (3): 299–304. McCintyre, R.S. *et al.*, 'Valproate, bipolar disorder and polycystic ovarian syndrome', *Bipolar Disord.* 2003 Feb; 5 (1): 28–35
2. 'Depression, anxiety and quality of life scores in seniors after an endurance exercise program', *Rev Bras Psiquiatr.* 2005 Dec; 27 (4): 266–71
3. Nowak, G. *et al.*, 'Zinc and depression. An update', *Pharmacol Rep.* 2005 Nov–Dec; 57 (6): 713–8

CHAPTER 18: GETTING THE EMOTIONAL SUPPORT YOU WANT

1. Yilmaz, M. *et al.*, 'Glucose intolerance, insulin resistance and cardiovascular risk factors in first degree relatives of women with polycystic ovary syndrome', *Hum Reprod.* 2005 Sep; 20 (9): 2414–20. Legro, R.S. *et al.*, 'Insulin resistance in the sisters of women with polycystic ovary syndrome: association with hyperandrogenemia rather than menstrual irregularity', *J Clin Endocrinol Metab.* 2002 May; 87 (5): 2128–33. Sir-Petermann, T. *et al.*, 'Prevalence of Type II diabetes mellitus and insulin resistance in parents of women with polycystic ovary syndrome', *Diabetologia.* 2002 Jul; 45 (7): 959–64. Sam, S. *et al.*, 'Dyslipidemia and metabolic syndrome in the sisters of women with polycystic ovary syndrome', *J Clin Endocrinol Metab.* 2005 Aug; 90 (8): 4797–802

RESOURCES

USEFUL CONTACTS

Here are some of the most relevant contacts and websites if you want to find out more about PCOS in general or hook up with other women with PCOS. One the best things about websites is that they are international so you can get some great help, advice and information from any of the websites listed here, not just from organizations based in your country. If you do decide to write to an organization, always send a stamped addressed envelope, as many of these are charities run by volunteers.

After visiting your doctor and getting his or her advice, a PCOS support group should be your next port of call. Groups like Verity in the UK or PCOS Support in the US can put you in touch with a support group in your local area and also give you the advice, support, information, and understanding you need to make informed choices about PCOS and your health and well-being.

USEFUL WEBSITES

PCOS

www.verity-pcos.org.uk

www.pcosupport.org – US PCOS support group website affiliated to Verity in the UK

www.posaa.asn.au – Australian support group website

www.pcosupport.org/pcoteen/about.html – PCOTeen is a division of PCOSA for women in their teens with PCOS

www.pcos.net – 'Helping women with PCOS' is the motto of this friendly US website which includes info on low-carb diets and ongoing research

www.pcos-equality.org.uk – Campaign group set up by women to fight the 'postcode lottery' that exists in the UK when applying for laser treatment for excess hair

www.soulcysters.com – US based e-group for women with PCOS to meet and exchange information

www.pcolist.org/mailman/listinfo/thincysters – US based e-group for cysters within the normal weight range.

www.ovarian-cysts-pcos.com/ Natural health solutions for women with PCOS

COMPLEMENTARY AND ALTERNATIVE MEDICINE

www.bcma.co.uk

http://nccam.nih.gov

www.internethealthlibrary.com

www.bloom.com.au

GLYCAEMIC INDEX

www.glycaemicindex.com

Information on the glycaemic index of foods, latest GI data, books and testing services

www.gidiet.com

A detailed guide to the GI diet, which also offers you the opportunity to submit any of your experiences with the GI diet and any tips, suggestions or recipes

Additional information and values for Glycaemic Index and

Glycaemic Load can be found at
www.glycaemicindex.com and
http://www.mendosa.com/
gilists.htm

DIABETES
www.diabetes.org
www.diabetes.org.uk
www.mendosa.com/org.htm
Amazing website which links you to
every other useful website on
diabetes/insulin resistance

**HEART
HEALTH/HYPERTENSION**
www.bcs.com
www.bhf.org.uk
www.hyp.ac.uk/bhsinfo
www.familyheart.org
www.americanheart.org

MIND/BODY/SPIRIT HEALING
www.kindredspirit.co.uk
http://peoplesmed.org/links.html
www.drweil.com/u/Events/

NUTRITION
www.eatright.org
www.thefooddoctor.o.uk
www.naturopathic.org
www.patrickholford.com

THYROID
www.thyroiduk.org
www.thyroid.com

WOMEN'S HEALTH
www.obgyn.net
www.nlm.nih.gov
www.healthywoman.org
www.whas.com.au

UK CONTACTS

PCOS
Verity
Unit AS20.01
The Aberdeen Centre
22–24 Highbury Grove
London N5 2EA
www.verity-pcos.org.uk
Verity has loads of information and
advice for women with PCOS, details
of events and other items of news.

COMPLEMENTARY THERAPIES

British Complementary Medicine Association
St Charles Hospital
Exmoor Street
London W10 6DZ
0208 964 1205

Council for Complementary and Alternative Medicine
179 Gloucester Place
London NW1 6DX
0207 724 9103

COUNSELLING/DEPRESSION

Psycho-educational support group for women with PCOS
Alexandra Cross and Rachel Green
Health Psychology Service
St Ann's Hospital
St Ann's Road
London N15 3TH
0208 442 6124
alexandra.cross@beh-mht.nhs.uk

The Samaritans
24-hour helpline: 0845 790 9090

British Association for Counselling
1 Regent Place
Rugby
Warwickshire CV21 2PJ

MIND – Mental Health Charity
15–19 Broadway
London E15 4BQ
0845 766 0163

DIABETES

Diabetes UK
10 Parkway
London NW1 7AA
0207 424 1000

DIET AND NUTRITION

British Dietetic Association
5th Floor, Charles House
148–149 Great Charles Street
Birmingham B3 3HT
0121 200 8080

British Nutrition Foundation
High Holborn House
52 High Holborn
London WC1V 6RQ
0207 404 6504

Vegetarian Society
Parkdale
Denham Road
Altrincham
Cheshire WA14 4QS
0161 928 0793

Vegan Society
Donald Watson House
7 Battle Road
St Leonards on Sea
East Sussex TN3 7AA
01424 427 393

EATING DISORDERS

Eating Disorders Association
103 Prince of Wales Road
Norfolk NR1 1DW
0845 634 1414

Overeaters Anonymous
01273 624 712
Nationwide local groups throughout
the UK

HEART HEALTH

British Heart Foundation
14 Fitzhardinge Street
London W1H 4DH
0207 388 0903

SUPPLEMENTS

Biocare Nutritional Supplements
0121 433 3727

The Herbalists' Centre
0207 935 0405

The Nutri Centre
0207 436 5122

Solgar Vitamins
01442 890355

Lambert Healthcare
01892 552120

Specialist Herbal Supplies
01273 202401

Higher Nature Ltd
01435 882880

WOMEN'S HEALTH

Women's Health
52 Featherstone Street
London EC1Y 8RT
0207 251 6580

Smoking Quitline
NHS helpline 0800 1690169

US CONTACTS

PCOS

Polycystic Ovarian Syndrome Association Inc, PCOSA
PO Box 80517
Portland, OR 97280
www.pcosupport.org
PCOSA is the US-based self-help group to which Verity in the UK is affiliated. A treasure trove of information, advice, help and support.

COMPLEMENTARY/ALTERNATIVE THERAPIES

National Clearing House for Complementary and Alternative Medicine
PO Box 8218
Silver Spring, MD 20907-8218
1-888-664-6226

COUNSELLING/DEPRESSION

Concerned Counselling
Telephone counselling service toll-free within the US: 1-888-415-8255

National Foundation for Depressive Illness
PO Box 2257
New York, NY 10016
212 268 4260

DIABETES

American Diabetes Association
1701 North Beauregard Street
Alexandria, VA 22311

DIET AND NUTRITION

The American Dietetic Association
216 West Jackson Boulevard
Chicago, IL 60606 6995
312 899 0040

Food and Nutrition Information Center
National Agriculture Library
10301 Baltimore Avenue
Room 304
Beltsville, MD 20705-2351
301 504 5719

North American Vegetarian Society
P.O. Box 72Q
Dolgeville, NY 13329
518-568-7970

American Vegan Society
56 Dinshah Lane
PO Box 369
Malaga, NJ 08328
856-694-2887

EATING DISORDERS

American Anorexia/Bulimia Association
418E 76th Street
New York, NY 10021
(212) 734 1114

HEART DISEASE

The American Heart Association
7272 Greenville Avenue
Dallas, TX 75231
214 762 6300
(also provides information about hypertension)

SUPPLEMENTS

Blessed Herbs
(800) 489 4372

Herbal Magic Inc
(415) 488 9488

Herbal Pharmacy
(541) 846 6262

May Way Trading
(510) 208 3113

Metagenics

(800) 692 9400

Nature's Apothecary

(303) 581 0288

Uni Key Health Systems

800 888 4353

International Academy of Compounding Pharmacists

(713) 933 8400 – will help you locate a local pharmacy that specializes in natural prescriptions

WOMEN'S HEALTH

National Women's Health Resource Centre NWHRC

120 Albany Street

Suite 820

New Brunswick, NJ 08901

877 986 9742

National clearing-house for information, internet links and resources about women's health

AUSTRALIAN CONTACTS

PCOS

Posaa – Polycystic Ovary Syndrome Association Of Australia

PO Box E140

Emerton

NSW 2770

612 4733 4342

www.posaa.asn.au

DIABETES

Diabetes Australia

AVA House

5/7 Phipps place

Deakin

ACT 2600

616 285 3277

WOMEN'S HEALTH

Women's Health Statewide

64 Pennington Terrace

Nth Adelaide SA 5006

08 8267 5366

FURTHER READING

PCOS

Colette Harris and Dr Adam Carey. *PCOS: A Woman's Guide to Dealing with Polycystic Ovary Syndrome* (Thorsons)
Colette Harris and Theresa Cheung. *The PCOS Diet Book* (Thorsons)
————. *The PCOS Protection Plan* (Hay House)
————. *PCOS and your Fertility* (Hay House)
Dr Samuel Thatcher. *PCOS: The Hidden Epidemic* (Perspectives Press)

BODY IMAGE

Tracy Gaudet. *Consciously Female*
Barbara Harris and Angela Hynes. *Shape Your Life: Four Weeks to a Better Body and a Better Life* (Hay House)
Marcia Hutchinson. *200 Ways to Love the Body You Have* (Crossing)

COMPLEMENTARY/ALTERNATIVE/HERBAL MEDICINE/MIND, BODY AND SPIRIT HEALING

Kitty Campion. *HolisticWomen's Herbal* (Bloomsbury)

Susan Clarke. *What ReallyWorks: The Insiders Guide to Natural Health* (Thorsons)

Tori Hudson. *Women's Encyclopedia of Natural Medicine* (McGraw Hill)

Deborah Keston. *Feeding the Body, nourishing the Soul* (Conari, 1997)

DETOX

Sandra Cabot. *The Liver Cleansing Diet* (Women's Health Advisory Service)

Ann Louise Gittleman. *The Living Beauty Detox Programme* (Harper San Francisco)

Amanda Ursell. *CleanseYour System* (Thorsons)

DIABETES

Rudy Bilous. *Understanding Diabetes* (British Medical Association)

Vern Cherewatenko and Paul Perry. *The Diabetes Cure* (Thorsons)

Milton Hammerly. *Diabetes — how to combine the best of traditional and alternative therapies* (Adams Media)

Annette Maggi and Jackie Boucher. *What you can do to prevent diabetes* (Wiley)

EATING DISORDERS

Carolyn Costin. *The Eating Disorder Sourcebook* (McGraw Hill)
Jane Hirshmann and Carol Munter. *When Women Stop Hating Their Bodies –*
Freeing Yourself from Food and Weight Obsession (Ballantine)
Richard Oakes-Ash. *Good Girls Do Swallow* (Mainstream Publishing)

ENDOMETRIOSIS

Dian Shepperson Mills and Michael Vernon. *Endometriosis – A Key to Healing*
through Nutrition (Thorsons)

FATIGUE

Erica White. *The Beat Fatigue Handbook* (Thorsons)

FITNESS

Rosemary Conley Fitness videos, BBC Worldwide and Video Collection,
Inc VHS
Sally Gunnell. *Be Your Best* (Thorsons)
Howard Kent. *The Complete Illustrated Guide to Yoga* (Element)

FOOD AND MOOD

Amanda Geary. *The Food and Mood Handbook* (Thorsons)

GIVING UP SMOKING

Allen Carr's Easy Way to Stop Smoking (Penguin)

Susannah Hayward. *Breathe Easy — The Friendly Stop Smoking Guide for Women* (Penguin)

HEALTHY EATING

Jean Carper. *Food — Your Miracle Medicine* (Simon and Schuster)

Theresa Cheung. *Living with the Glycaemic Factor* (Sheldon)

Maurice Hansen and Jill Marsden. *E is for Additives* (Thorsons)

Anthony Leeds. *The GI Factor* (Hodder and Stoughton)

Gillian McKeith. *You Are What You Eat* (Penguin)

HEART HEALTH/HYPERTENSION

Chris Davidson. *Understanding Coronary Heart Disease* (British Medical Association)

Sara Rosenthal. *50 Ways Women can Prevent Heart Disease* (Lowell House)

INSULIN RESISTANCE

Jack Challem. *Syndrome X: Complete Nutritional Programme for Insulin Resistance* (John Wiley)

Cheryl Hart. *The Insulin Resistance Diet* (McGraw Hill)

ORGANIC LIVING

Lynda Brown. *Organic Living – Simple Strategies for a Better Life*
Karen Sullivan. *Organic Living in 10 Simple Lessons* (Barnes Ed)

RECIPES

Nadine Abensur. *Crank's Bible* (Orion)
Louise Blair. *Low GI Cookbook: 80 Recipes to Help You Lose Weight and Gain Health* (Hamlyn)
Nigel Denby. *The GL Diet Cookbook* (Thorsons)
Patrick Holford. *Holford Low GI Diet Cookbook* (Piatkus)

STRESS/SELF-ESTEEM/LIFE SKILLS

David Burns. *10 Days to Great Self-esteem* (Vermillion)
Louise Hay. *Affirmations for Self-Esteem* (Hay House)
Robert Holden. *Stressbusters* (Thorsons)
Phil McGraw. *Life Strategies* (Free Press)
Matthew McKay. *Self-Esteem Companion* (New Harbinger)
Jeffrey Young and Janet Klosko. *Reinventing Your Life*

SUPPLEMENTS

James and Phyliss Balch. *Prescription for Nutritional Healing* (Avery)
Patrick Holford. *The Optimum Nutrition Bible* (Piatkus)
Linda Lazarides. *The Nutritional Health Bible* (Thorsons)
Earl Mindel's Supplement Bible (Thorsons)

THYROID

Martin Budd. *Why Am I so Tired? Is Your Thyroid Making You Ill?* (Thorsons)

WEIGHT LOSS

Pete Cohen and Judith Verity. *Lighten Up* (Century)
Phil McGraw. *The Ultimate Weight Solution* (Free Press)
Barry Sears. *The Zone — A Dietary Road Map to Lose Weight Permanently* (Harper Collins)

WELL WOMAN

Joan Borysenko. *A Woman's Book of Life* (Riverhead Books)
Marilyn Glenville. *The Natural Health Handbook for Women* (Piatkus)
Christiane Northrup. *Women's Bodies, Women's Wisdom* (Bantam)

INDEX